Terenure Branch Tel. 4907035

Irish Pregnancy

Terenure Branch Tel. 4907035

A Guide for Expectant Mothers

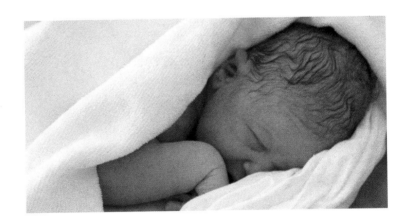

Dr Peter Boylan MAO FRCPI FRCOG

National Maternity Hospital

The O'Brien Press

This revised edition first published in 2015 by
The O'Brien Press Limited,
12 Terenure Road East, Rathgar, Dublin 6, D06 HD27, Ireland
Tel: +353 1 4923333; Fax: +353 1 4922777
E-mail: books@obrien.ie
Website: www.obrien.ie

ISBN: 978-1-84717-814-5

Originally published in 2005 by A. & A. Farmar Ltd
Revised editions published in 2006, 2008 and 2012

5 4 3 2 1
19 18 17 16 15

Photographs courtesy of Corbis (p. 107), Fotosearch (p. 110), Imagefile
(p. 77, 130, 153, 165), all others of the National Maternity Hospital

Text and cover design by Kevin Gurry
Drawings by Alice Campbell
Index and text setting by Bookworks

Printed and bound in Poland by Białostockie Zakłady Graficzne S.A.
The paper in this book is produced using pulp from managed forests.

acknowledgements

Many people helped in the production of this book, but a few deserve special mention and thanks. Laura George was very helpful in the early stages and gave generously of her time, expertise as a journalist, and practical experience as a mother. Midwives Margaret Fanagan, who runs the antenatal education classes in the National Maternity Hospital, and Margaret Hanahoe, who coordinates the National Maternity Hospital home birth and Domino schemes, read the script and made useful suggestions and corrections. I am most grateful for their assistance. My editor, Anna Farmar, showed great patience and faith in the project from the beginning. Putting pen to paper is only the beginning, the editing and production of the text are hugely important and without Anna's skills you would not be holding this book in your hands.

I am also grateful to my colleagues who answered my many question with customary grace and good humour. Finally, I have to record my gratitude to all the mothers whose lively interest in their pregnancies was the stimulus to writing this guide.

This latest edition (2015) has been updated to reflect recent developments in obstetric care.

I have made every effort to ensure that all the information in the book is both accurate and up to date. Any errors or omissions are entirely my responsibility.

Dr Peter Boylan
July 2015

contents

introduction

I have been privileged to observe and participate in many thousands of pregnancies and births over more than thirty years as a practising obstetrician. Each birth was unique and each was an awesome experience.

Over the years I have perceived the need for a reliable, up to date source of information to answer the many questions that arise during pregnancy. Often the answers are needed at a time when the doctor or midwife are not available, for example at weekends, on holidays, at night, or in between antenatal visits—this book will help to fill that gap.

Although each pregnancy is unique there are common themes to all and similar questions come up for most mothers and couples: Will I have a miscarriage? What's causing that cramp in my tummy? Will our baby be all right? Will I be able to deliver my baby? Will I need a caesarean? If you have the answers to some of your questions before your visits to the doctor or midwife you will be able to get more value from the visits. You could, for example, use the opportunity to confirm your understanding of a particular situation or indeed expand on your understanding. More knowledge about what is happening during your pregnancy will hopefully lessen any fears you may have and make the whole experience even more rewarding.

I hope I have covered all the relevant issues. The book is not meant to be totally comprehensive, answering every possible query that might arise, particularly about possible abnormal development of the baby. What I have tried to do is to provide the information that in my experience most mothers-to-be look for. This latest edition reflects recent developments in obstetric care.

In the Ireland of today the majority of pregnancies and births are uncomplicated and result in a healthy mother and baby. This book will, I hope, help make the whole event a more enjoyable experience.

Dr Peter Boylan
July 2015

1 becoming pregnant

Pregnancy marks an exciting new phase in your life. Very soon after conception—within days—your body will begin to undergo profound changes as the embryo starts to develop and pregnancy hormones kick in.

Pregnancy actually begins when the sperm penetrates the outer layer of the ovum (egg) to cause fertilisation and the conception of a child. This process usually takes place in the fallopian tube, which connects the uterus to the ovary. For most women the first sign of pregnancy is a missed period. A pregnancy test, available from chemists, will give a positive result within days of your being late or even before you miss a period.

How you get pregnant

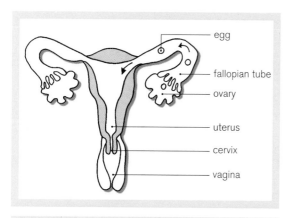

egg

fallopian tube

ovary

uterus

cervix

vagina

OVULATION

Every month one or two eggs are released from one (or both) of your ovaries. The egg is wafted into your fallopian tube and on into your uterus.

Ovulation

Each month, in the middle of your menstrual cycle, one or two eggs are ejected from your ovaries where they have been since before you were born. This process is called ovulation.

Following ovulation, the egg sticks to the surface of the ovary, surrounded by a layer of cells that attract the open end of the fallopian tube. The fallopian tubes' finger-like projections sweep across the surface and collect the egg from it. Once in the tube, the egg is wafted towards the uterus by other fine finger-like projections (cilia), which beat in the direction of the uterus. If it is not fertilised the lining of the uterus comes away in your menstrual flow, your period. For you to get pregnant the egg needs to be fertilised by sperm.

Fertilisation

With each act of intercourse, between 200 and 300 million sperm are deposited in the vagina. Only a small proportion of these (less than 200) actually get anywhere near the egg. The rest either drain from the vagina or are killed by hostile conditions in the vagina, cervix or uterus. The heartiest sperm gain entry to the fallopian tube within 5 minutes of ejaculation and are helped on their journey by involuntary contractions of the uterus and the dipping motion of the cervix during female orgasm, although orgasm is not necessary for fertilisation to occur. They can survive for up to 72 hours so that intercourse does not have to be timed precisely in relation to ovulation. Once in the vicinity of an egg, the sperm undergoes a process known as capacitation, which involves a series of chemical and structural changes that make it fertile and enable it to penetrate the egg's outer shell.

Fertilisation usually takes place in the middle of the fallopian tube.

At fertilisation, there is a complex splitting of the genetic material from the sperm and egg respectively so that the new embryo takes half its complement of genes from each parent. The process of fertilisation is so dramatic and complex that it can be likened to the 'big bang' at the beginning of the universe.

After fertilisation, it takes 8–13 days for the developing embryo to implant in the wall of the womb, or uterus, and another several days before the embryo starts drawing nutrients from your bloodstream, by which time you will probably be aware you are pregnant.

A couple with no fertility problems have a 25–30 per cent chance of achieving fertilisation in each unprotected cycle where intercourse occurs at the fertile time. However, only about 50 per cent of resulting embryos successfully lodge in the wall of the uterus and develop into a healthy baby. A significant proportion are lost during normal menstruation; others implant and fail to develop, coming away with the menstrual flow. In these circumstances, most women do not even know they were 'pregnant' during that particular cycle although

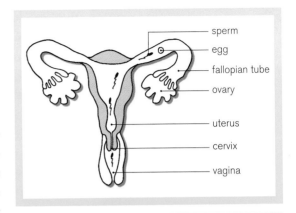

BEFORE FERTILISATION
Up to 300 million sperm enter your vagina during intercourse. Only a few will get as far as the egg in the fallopian tube and only one will be successful in penetrating the egg's outer layer and fertilising it.

not just the baby
The fertilised egg will develop into the baby, the placenta, the umbilical cord and the amniotic fluid (waters) contained by the membranes.

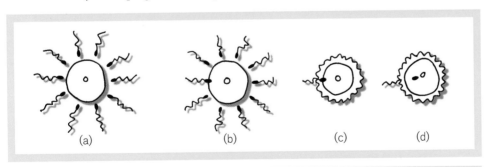

FERTILISATION
(a) The few sperm that have survived as far as the fallopian tube surround the egg.
(b) One sperm gains entry.
(c) The egg develops a protective layer to prevent other sperm from entering.
(d) The egg is now fertilised and the process of cell division begins.

home pregnancy testing

Taking a test is extremely easy. You simply pee onto the swab provided and wait as per the instructions on the kit. A result shows up in the testing window. Tests are usually extremely accurate in the days following a missed period. A positive result is never wrong, although a negative result may occur because you have taken the test too early. Most women end up taking more than one test, either to reassure themselves that their test result is indeed positive or because a test result is negative and they want to retest a few days later.

they may have a slightly heavier period than normal. Some women, however, are acutely sensitive to changes in their bodies and are aware within hours of fertilisation that they have become pregnant.

The fertile period

The most fertile time of your cycle is the few days immediately preceding ovulation. In an average 28-day cycle (where day 1 is considered the first day of the period), ovulation occurs on day 14, with menstruation beginning 14 days later. In this cycle, the most fertile window is between days 12–16 because no matter how long an individual's cycle runs, menstruation usually starts 14 days after ovulation. To estimate ovulation, simply count backwards 14 days from the day your next period is expected (thus in a 35-day cycle, ovulation occurs on day 21). Obviously, a woman with a long cycle ovulates less frequently during the year than a woman with an average length cycle. Many women get a pain in the lower abdomen at the time of ovulation and so can tell when they ovulate.

Many couples who are trying to conceive make the mistake of waiting to have sex until they feel the woman has already ovulated. This may be too late. It is better that the sperm be on their way to intercept the egg prior to ovulation, so that the single fertilising sperm is already there when the egg is on its downward journey through the fallopian tube. The sperm have time on their side and can wait. Their normal life span is 48–72 hours, whereas an egg only lasts about 24 hours.

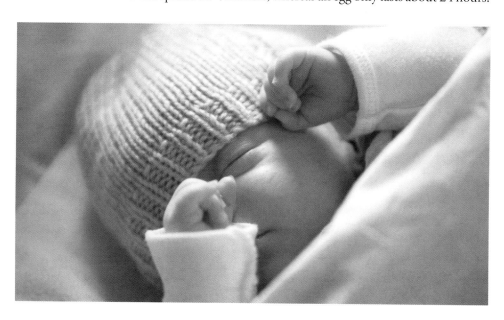

The reason why the fertile period is described as including the two days on either side of ovulation is because the precise day of ovulation often varies by a day or two from one cycle to the next. An ovulation kit identifies the day of ovulation in a given cycle and so is probably advisable if you are experiencing difficulty in conceiving.

Menstrual history chart

If you are planning a pregnancy, you should note in your diary the first day of your periods for two reasons. First, good records will make calculating your fertile window easier. If your cycles are at all irregular, you may be able to see a pattern in the chart that will help you predict your fertile times more accurately. Secondly, if you do get pregnant, your pregnancy will be dated from the first day of your last menstrual period even though fertilisation does not occur until approximately two weeks later. When we say a woman is 16 weeks pregnant, it means that it has been 16 weeks since the first day of her last period.

Ann's menstrual chart shows she has a 29-day cycle on average (it is anywhere from 27–32 days long). Therefore, she can expect to ovulate approximately 15 days after her period begins. (Although in February it turned out she ovulated two days later because she had one of her longer cycles, and in March she ovulated a day earlier because she had one of her shorter cycles.)

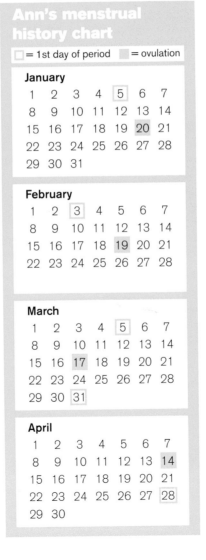

Ann's menstrual history chart

☐ = 1st day of period   ▢ = ovulation

January
1 2 3 4 5 6 7
8 9 10 11 12 13 14
15 16 17 18 19 20 21
22 23 24 25 26 27 28
29 30 31

February
1 2 3 4 5 6 7
8 9 10 11 12 13 14
15 16 17 18 19 20 21
22 23 24 25 26 27 28

March
1 2 3 4 5 6 7
8 9 10 11 12 13 14
15 16 17 18 19 20 21
22 23 24 25 26 27 28
29 30 31

April
1 2 3 4 5 6 7
8 9 10 11 12 13 14
15 16 17 18 19 20 21
22 23 24 25 26 27 28
29 30

when is my fertile period?

Fill in your own details opposite by underlining the days of your period. When your next period starts, count back 14 days from the first day of your period to get the date of probable ovulation for the month gone by. Circle it, the two days preceding it, and the two days after. This is your fertile period. Now you can see if there's a discrepancy between when you thought you would ovulate and when you probably did. If there is a difference between the two dates you should consider buying a test ovulation kit to find out exactly when you ovulate rather than trying to second guess your body.

home ovulation prediction

Kits are available from most chemists and are a quick and easy way of determining the most fertile days of your cycle. During a normal menstrual cycle, the level of luteinising hormone (LH) surges just before ovulation occurs. A simple urine test tells whether the hormone is present in significant amounts. Results are usually indicated by a simple colour change on the test swab or by the appearance of a blue line in the testing window, depending on the type of kit chosen.

your menstrual history chart

January
```
1   2   3   4   5   6   7
8   9   10  11  12  13  14
15  16  17  18  19  20  21
22  23  24  25  26  27  28
29  30  31
```

February
```
1   2   3   4   5   6   7
8   9   10  11  12  13  14
15  16  17  18  19  20  21
22  23  24  25  26  27  28
```

March
```
1   2   3   4   5   6   7
8   9   10  11  12  13  14
15  16  17  18  19  20  21
22  23  24  25  26  27  28
29  30  31
```

April
```
1   2   3   4   5   6   7
8   9   10  11  12  13  14
15  16  17  18  19  20  21
22  23  24  25  26  27  28
29  30
```

May
```
1   2   3   4   5   6   7
8   9   10  11  12  13  14
15  16  17  18  19  20  21
22  23  24  25  26  27  28
29  30  31
```

June
```
1   2   3   4   5   6   7
8   9   10  11  12  13  14
15  16  17  18  19  20  21
22  23  24  25  26  27  28
29  30
```

July
```
1   2   3   4   5   6   7
8   9   10  11  12  13  14
15  16  17  18  19  20  21
22  23  24  25  26  27  28
29  30  31
```

August
```
1   2   3   4   5   6   7
8   9   10  11  12  13  14
15  16  17  18  19  20  21
22  23  24  25  26  27  28
29  30  31
```

September
```
1   2   3   4   5   6   7
8   9   10  11  12  13  14
15  16  17  18  19  20  21
22  23  24  25  26  27  28
29  30
```

October
```
1   2   3   4   5   6   7
8   9   10  11  12  13  14
15  16  17  18  19  20  21
22  23  24  25  26  27  28
29  30  31
```

November
```
1   2   3   4   5   6   7
8   9   10  11  12  13  14
15  16  17  18  19  20  21
22  23  24  25  26  27  28
29  30
```

December
```
1   2   3   4   5   6   7
8   9   10  11  12  13  14
15  16  17  18  19  20  21
22  23  24  25  26  27  28
29  30  31
```

How long should it take?

A perfectly normal, healthy couple having regular intercourse can take up to a year to become pregnant. Eighty per cent of couples conceive within the first year of trying; 90 per cent conceive within two years.

A home test will confirm that pregnancy has begun and then you can begin to adapt your lifestyle to the demands of pregnancy.

Unplanned pregnancy

If you haven't been trying to conceive, and discover you are pregnant, you may be concerned that you did not alter your lifestyle appropriately in the very early stages of pregnancy. As long as you are healthy and are not addicted to any substances, it is extremely unlikely that you have put your baby at risk of not developing properly, even if you have not made any major adjustments to your lifestyle.

Learning that you are pregnant can be a tremendous shock, even if the pregnancy is planned. If it is unplanned, your situation is more complex. Confidential counselling, free of charge, is available to anyone who needs it. Ask your GP for a referral or contact:
+OPTIONS 1850 62 26 26
www.positiveoptions.ie

Preparing for pregnancy

If you are hoping to become pregnant there are a few things you can and should do to improve your general health and so help your pregnancy to progress smoothly. Most pregnancies are not planned, however, and still progress normally, resulting in a healthy mother and baby.

Get physically fit

Generally speaking, women who are physically fit have easier pregnancies and births. Pregnancy places a lot of physiological demands on your body. For example, your blood volume rapidly increases by 40 per cent, your hormone levels surge, and your body ligaments become soft and loosen under the influence of pregnancy hormones. (This looseness accounts for many of the aches and pains associated with later pregnancy.) Since you should not start a demanding new fitness programme once you are pregnant, the time to act is before conception. Getting ready to have a baby is as good a reason as any to make healthy lifestyle changes.

Watch your weight

You should try not to be too overweight when you conceive—the extra weight gained during pregnancy is hard enough to shift without having even more to worry about. Women who are markedly overweight when they conceive are at increased risk of developing diabetes during pregnancy. In addition, if you are very overweight, it will be more difficult for your carers to scan and feel the baby to check its progress, and labour and delivery will be more difficult for you.

it takes two

There is increasing evidence that paternal health at the time of conception matters. As you prepare for pregnancy by exercising, eating a good diet, limiting alcohol intake and stopping smoking, your partner may wish to lend more than just moral support and jump on the bandwagon with you . . . after all, the baby will inherit 50 per cent of his genes too.

Weight gain in pregnancy comes from two sources: what you eat, and the pregnancy. The pregnancy includes your baby, the placenta, growth of the uterus, increase in blood volume, increase in breast size and fluid retention—an average weight gain of 10–15 kg (20–30 lb). Only what you eat is under your control. Therefore, if you eat a good balanced diet, any weight you put on during the pregnancy can be attributed to your pregnancy and will be lost within a few months of the birth. However, if you eat junk food you will put on excessive weight, whether you are pregnant or not. The amount of weight you gain in pregnancy bears no relationship to your baby's size. This is why many obstetricians do not weigh women on a regular basis during pregnancy.

Take folic acid supplements

In terms of specifics, folic acid supplementation is the only factor in a woman's diet that has been shown conclusively to improve a baby's chances of being born healthy. It is particularly important for women who have previously had a baby with a neural tube defect such as spina bifida, or anencephaly. If you fall into this category, you should begin supplementation (5 mg/day) two months before conception and continue taking it for the first twelve weeks of pregnancy. This will not eliminate the risk, but will reduce the chance of recurrence by more than two-thirds. For women who have not previously had an affected baby, there is good evidence that a multivitamin preparation containing a much lower dose of folic acid (0.4 mg/day) protects against neural tube defects and indeed all other congenital malformations apart from cleft lip and/or palate. If you didn't know about these supplements before getting pregnant, or forget to take them, don't worry. Only a small percentage of women actually take supplements before pregnancy and the vast majority have no problems. Spina bifida is a rare occurrence, even without pre-pregnancy folic acid and multivitamin supplementation.

a healthy embryo grows from one single cell and develops at a breathtaking rate. The process of division and recombination of chromosomes is so intricate that a variety of problems may arise. These range from failure of the embryo to develop at all (early miscarriage) to serious conditions in the developing baby, which may cause death or varying degrees of disability or abnormality. In some cases, the abnormality may only become apparent when the affected individual becomes involved in reproduction, as either a mother or father.

Don't smoke

You should not smoke before, during or after pregnancy. Smoking is directly harmful to your own health, causing lung cancer and other chronic respiratory conditions like emphysema and bronchitis. It also predisposes you to other types of cancer, such as cancer of the cervix. Smoking affects your and your partner's fertility adversely and thus can make conception more difficult. Once you are pregnant, smoking reduces both food and oxygen supply to your baby, so give up now. Finally, smoking may result in the premature birth of your baby and low birth weight. Your partner should also refrain from smoking. Smoking affects sperm viability and passive smoking can be harmful to you.

Don't drink too much

Heavy drinking can reduce male sperm count; prolonged excessive drinking can harm a developing foetus. Both of you should moderate your alcoholic intake when trying to get pregnant. Don't worry if you have been drinking moderately in the early stages of pregnancy, as it appears that you would need to be drinking heavily throughout pregnancy to harm your baby.

Check your medication

Certain drugs prescribed for particular illnesses or ongoing conditions may be associated with or directly cause abnormality in a developing foetus, for example, retinoic acid (Roaccutane) or tetracycline antibiotics for skin acne. If you are taking medication, it is wise to check with the prescribing physician or obstetrician regarding their continued use while you are trying to conceive and during pregnancy. It may be that the dosage or type of medication needs alteration before pregnancy. Some drugs may even act as incidental contraceptives. Never stop taking any medication without consulting your doctor first. Medications taken for the control of epilepsy and for depression are particularly important.

Ensure you are immune to rubella

If you are contemplating pregnancy you should ensure that you are immune to rubella (German measles) because contracting this disease during pregnancy, particularly in the early stages, may cause significant damage to the developing foetus. The risk to the baby appears to reduce sharply after 16 weeks of pregnancy. In most Western societies, immunisation is offered to all schoolchildren and congenital rubella is extremely rare as a result. However, immunity may disappear later, so it is best to check your immunity before trying for a baby. All pregnant women are routinely tested for rubella and if found not to be immune are offered immunisation immediately following pregnancy, before they conceive again.

the influence of genes

How our bodies develop is determined by the way our inherited genes are distributed, how they mix and interact. Thus the nature of your embryo is determined by the genes it inherits at the moment of conception. The process is completely outside anyone's control and explains the wide variety of appearance, personality traits and talents among children of the same parents. There is no evidence that time of cycle, position during intercourse or side from which ovulation occurs have any influence on gender or future development.

Find out if you have had chickenpox

Try to find out before you get pregnant whether or not you have had chickenpox because it has the potential to harm the baby in early pregnancy. A routine blood test will show if you have had the disease; in that case your baby will be completely protected. If you have not had chickenpox you should avoid children with the disease while you are trying to get pregnant and for the first 12–14 weeks of pregnancy.

If you are over 35

More women than ever are having babies later, although physically the optimal time to be pregnant is in your twenties. Unfortunately, after the age of 35, the risks associated with pregnancy do increase, regardless of how young you feel. There is a slightly increased risk of high blood pressure and diabetes in pregnancy for women over 35 and a higher incidence of random (i.e. not inherited) chromosomal disorders such as Down syndrome in babies born to women over 35. For this reason also the chances of miscarriage increase gradually with advancing maternal age.

Although the risk of a random chromosomal abnormality increases with advancing maternal age, the risk is lower than most people expect and there is a gradual, rather than sudden, increase in the chance of such an occurrence. Even at the age of 40, you have only a 1 per cent chance of having a baby with Down syndrome.

Genetic counselling

Genetic counselling before pregnancy is generally not necessary unless there is a clearly identified inherited condition present in one of your families such as inherited Down syndrome. Such conditions are rare but if your family is affected ask your GP or gynaecologist to refer you to a genetic counsellor.

Have a cervical/pap smear

Every woman who is sexually active should have a cervical smear at least every three years. More frequent reviews may be required if there has been an abnormality in the past. If you have not had a cervical smear in the last two years, you should have one before embarking on pregnancy. Smear abnormalities are generally easily treated on an outpatient basis but may deteriorate if left untreated for a long time. A mildly abnormal smear can safely be reviewed after your pregnancy. Since treatment is more complicated during pregnancy and so is better avoided, it is best to confirm a normal smear before becoming pregnant.

your baby's sex will be determined by whether the fertilising sperm is male or female so it's always your partner who determines your child's sex.

When to stop contraception

There is no hard evidence to suggest that hormonal contraceptives (the pill, Depo-provera injections) taken in early pregnancy (for example, if a woman is unaware she is pregnant) are harmful to the early developing embryo. It is safe to attempt conception in the first month after stopping the pill as the amount of hormones in modern preparations is very small and is quickly eliminated from the body. Likewise, failure of the morning after pill does not appear to influence an ongoing pregnancy or harm a developing a baby in any way.

The coil, or IUCD (intrauterine contraceptive device), on the other hand, is associated with an increased risk of ectopic pregnancy (pregnancy in the fallopian tube) and miscarriage or very premature delivery. Clearly, the coil should be removed prior to a planned pregnancy. If you conceive with a coil in the uterus, it can be visualised on ultrasound, allowing a decision to be taken on whether or not it should be removed. If the threads are visible on vaginal examination it is usually removed. If the doctor can't see it, it will be left in place and usually comes away at the time of delivery. It will not interfere with the development of your baby.

After a miscarriage

If you have just had a miscarriage, you may try to conceive again as soon as you feel emotionally and physically ready—there is no need to use contraceptives. If you become pregnant in the cycle immediately following a miscarriage you will not face increased risk of miscarriage in your new pregnancy. Each pregnancy is a completely separate event uninfluenced by previous pregnancies.

If however, miscarriage has occurred after eight weeks, a d&c (dilatation of the cervix and curettage) may be required to empty the uterus before attempting to get pregnant again.

General recommendations

- Eat a well-balanced, sensible diet
- Take folic acid (0.4 mg/day)
- Take a larger dose of folic acid (5 mg/day) if you have already had a baby with a neural tube defect
- Stop smoking
- Cut down, or stop, your drinking
- Check you are immune to rubella (German measles) and chickenpox
- Have a cervical smear test if you have not had one in the last two years
- Get reasonably fit
- Check with your doctor about whether you should continue with prescription medication

Frequently asked questions

I have diabetes. For how long must it be under control before I try to get pregnant?
At least three months—see your diabetic physician and consult an obstetrician prior to getting pregnant.

I have had three unexplained miscarriages. Should I consult my doctor before I try to conceive again?
Yes. It is important to investigate the possible causes of those miscarriages and rule out an identifiable cause for their recurrence. This may involve a blood test for both partners to rule out genetic problems and lupus antibodies. Identifiable causes are however quite rare so that the likelihood of getting an answer is really quite slim.

Are there any work hazards (x-rays, chemicals) that are potentially dangerous when trying to conceive?
Yes. Ideally, you should not have x-rays in the second half of your menstrual cycle, just in case you are already pregnant and don't know it yet. Exposure to high dose x-rays may harm your developing baby and cause miscarriage or predispose the baby to the development of leukemia in childhood. Low dose x-rays, such as dental x-rays, do not cause problems. It is difficult to give definitive advice regarding exposure to chemicals as there are so many possibilities. In general, it does not appear that normal safe work practices predispose to miscarriage or infertility. Fumes from paint appear to be harmless but nonetheless, make sure the area you are painting in is well ventilated—open the doors and windows.

My sister has a daughter with Down syndrome. Should I consider genetic counselling?
There are two types of Down's—the most common is a random occurrence but there is also a rare inherited type. Ask your sister which type her daughter has and if you are still concerned, ask your gynaecologist or GP for a referral to a genetic counsellor.

Should I stop smoking before I try to conceive?
Yes, doing so will increase your fertility and once you are pregnant you are advised to stop anyway. Smoking carries a higher risk of miscarriage and low birth weight.

I have three girls and desperately want to have a boy. Do any of the diets or high-tech treatments for influencing a baby's sex work?

Not to a sufficient degree to merit a considerable financial or emotional investment in them. With every pregnancy you have a 50/50 chance of having a baby of the sex you are hoping for, and existing diets and treatments do not improve this statistic dramatically. It is the fertilising sperm that determines the sex of your child, and millions of sperm are released each time you have intercourse. So choosing an X or Y sperm is not simple when there are so many.

Complex diets, which can always blame failure to produce the desired boy or girl on the patient's inability to follow the diet precisely, do not give impressive results. Remember, the sex of your baby is determined by its father: you will always produce an X chromosome no matter what diet you're on, whereas sperm are either X or Y. Undoubtedly, there will be major advances in this area in future, but in the meantime, it is wiser to conceive naturally.

I got pregnant over the Christmas holidays and drank a lot more then than I normally would because I didn't know I was pregnant yet. Will my baby be OK?

There is no evidence that heavy drinking very early in pregnancy causes any long-term harm or that it causes miscarriage. Once you are aware that you are pregnant you should restrict your alcohol intake to no more than one or two units a day.

What is pre-implantation diagnosis?

Pre-implantation diagnosis is a technique used in conjunction with IVF to determine if an embryo has an inherited condition, before it is placed in the mother's uterus. It is a form of very early antenatal diagnosis. A cell is taken from the very early developing embryo, following IVF, and analysed for the presence or absence of the condition. If the condition is not present the healthy embryo is placed in the mother's uterus, hopefully to go on and develop into a healthy baby. If the condition is present the embryo is not placed in the uterus. There is very limited avalability of pre-implantation diagnosis in Ireland. If you feel it may be relevant to you, ask your obstetrician.

2 hospital or home birth?

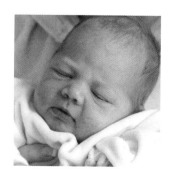

Once you know you are pregnant you should decide where you want to go for your antenatal care and for the delivery of your baby. Your first step is to visit your GP or family doctor to discuss what sort of care you wish to choose for your pregnancy and delivery. The main choices are between hospital and home or something in-between, where care is largely home-based but delivery is in hospital. There are many considerations to take into account when making your choice, but the main one should always be your own and your baby's health and safety.

Shared care: GP and hospital

Many GPs share care with the hospital and this is a very good choice. It enables your GP to be aware of how your pregnancy is progressing and facilitates the resolution of many of the minor problems you may encounter. If you have other children it is often more convenient to visit your GP's surgery rather than making the trek to hospital. Many GPs have midwives working with them also and this provides a ready source of information and care in an uncomplicated pregnancy. Attending a GP for the duration of your pregnancy should also help you develop a relationship with your GP which is helpful when you are bringing your new baby for immunisation etc. If you don't have a GP get one now! Looking after a new baby can sometimes be a daunting experience and a good local GP is an invaluable resource when your little one gets sick, as he or she inevitably will.

Hospital: public or private?

The best public care assigns you to a midwife/medical team at the antenatal stage so they can follow your pregnancy from beginning to end. Check what's on offer from the various hospitals in terms of continuity of care. While it is likely you will get the same standard of care whether you are a public or private patient, it is unlikely you will see the same doctor at every visit if you go public.

The semi-private option allows you to see the same doctor for antenatal care, a midwife attends the birth and your hospital stay can be in a semi-private ward.

If you go private you will be looked after by the specialist you have chosen for the duration of your pregnancy and the six weeks afterwards. A midwife looks after you in labour, in consultation with your doctor who attends for the delivery. This ease of access to your doctor is the major advantage of private care. Private health insurance will make

breaking the news

Many prospective parents delay telling friends and family their big news until the fourth month because most miscarriages occur in the first trimester (three months). Many parents delay telling their other children even longer as the wait can seem unbearably long to a child. However, in an age of instant gratification, it is a good idea to convey the true duration of pregnancy—a longer lead-in time gives everyone time to adjust to the idea of a new baby.

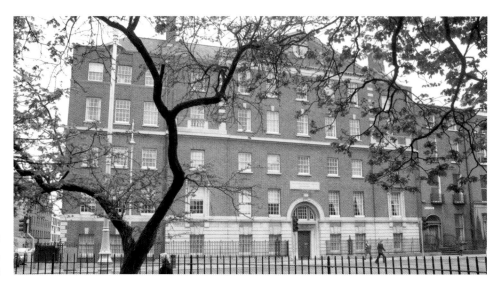

The National
Maternity Hospital,
Holles Street, Dublin

a contribution towards both hospital stay and your doctor's fees. You can ring your insurer directly to get exact figures if you are in doubt about your ability to afford private care.

The only other issue in the private versus public debate is having a private room. If you have had a difficult pregnancy or already have children, having a room of your own and some peace and quiet may be worth a premium. Wards can be very noisy and busy, day and night. This has both advantages and disadvantages. While it may be more difficult to rest when you want to due to other people's visitors and crying infants, some first-time mothers say that watching and talking to experienced mothers on the ward is invaluable in helping to get off to a good start.

Remember also that no hospital can guarantee you a private room and that such rooms are few and far between. The provision of private rooms is controlled by the Department of Health. In general they are not sympathetic to the provision of enough accommodation to meet the demand.

Choosing a doctor and hospital–if you are going private

- Ask friends and family who have had babies recently about their experiences—in detail. Did the doctor take time to answer questions? Was the doctor strict about weight gain? Did the doctor listen to the patient's preferences about pain relief, length of stay in hospital, induction when overdue, breastfeeding?
- Ask about the doctor's annual holidays and who covers in his or her absence.
- Ask about cover arrangements for weekends or if your doctor is unavailable for some reason. Remember, your baby may decide to come when your doctor has some unavoidable commitment—his or her own child's birthday party on a Sunday afternoon, for example!

Ask how many people share a room. If it's a priority for you, ask what is the likelihood of getting a private room?

Home birth

A planned home birth can be a hugely satisfying experience if all goes well, and provided proper planning and appropriate precautions are in place. But it's not for everyone. In most European countries home birth is an infrequent choice, partly because of lack of infrastructure to provide a safe and satisfactory service, and partly because of lack of demand. The decision to give birth at home is obviously not to be taken lightly, so you should research the pros and cons before you make your decision.

The main concern people have with home birth relates to safety. While problems are rare, the speed at which they can develop explains why so many experienced obstetricians are so unenthusiastic about home births. The birthing process can only be defined as perfectly normal in retrospect, after a baby is seen to be healthy and the mother has not suffered an unexpected haemorrhage or other unpredictable complication.

Home birth is suitable if:

- You have already delivered a baby vaginally, although it may be suitable on your first birth
- You have an uncomplicated pregnancy—no bleeding or high blood pressure or problems with the growth of the baby
- You are expecting only one baby (not twins)
- The baby is positioned head first (not breech)
- The baby is appropriately grown
- Labour starts spontaneously between 37 and 42 weeks
- The amniotic fluid is clear
- Labour progresses at a normal rate
- The foetal heart rate remains normal.
- You are happy to labour without pain relief.

For all concerned the primary objective is safety for both you and your baby. With this in mind it is really only sensible to plan for a home birth if your pregnancy is uncomplicated.

home or away

Advantages of home birth:
you are in your own home environment
you are not subject to hospital routine
you are near the rest of your family.

Advantages of hospital birth:
emergency services for you and your baby are on the spot
pain-relieving medications and epidurals are readily available
24-hour midwifery is provided
medical help is at hand while you are in hospital after the birth
your baby will probably be able to have the heel test and BCG vaccine done before you go home.

safe home birth

Within well-recognised boundaries, international experience has shown home birth to be safe. Many mothers who choose home birth have already had one birth in hospital but found the experience unsatisfying or the first birth difficult. You should remember when deciding where to have your baby second time around that if you delivered your first baby vaginally, no matter how difficult it was, it is unlikely to be as traumatic next time.

Home-based birth is not suitable if:

You have certain medical conditions, such as diabetes, high blood pressure, epilepsy, history of clots in the leg or lung, infections such as HIV

You lack family support or suitable facilities in the home

Your home is more than 25 minutes away by ambulance in rush hour traffic

You have gynaecological problems such as cervical incompetence, exposure to DES, fibroids or previous surgery for fibroids, or abnormalities of the uterus or vagina

You have had a caesarean section, severe pre-eclampsia, retained placenta on two occasions, haemorrhage

Previous pregnancies resulted in stillbirth or neonatal death, premature birth or shoulder dystocia.

You should be prepared to be flexible if a complication does arise during the pregnancy, or indeed labour. Your, and your baby's, best interests may be best served by transfer to hospital-based care. This doesn't mean you can't have a normal birth. If the problem is not too serious, for example a minor degree of anaemia at the end of pregnancy, there is no reason why you shouldn't have a normal birth in the hospital, cared for by the same midwife who would have been at your home for the birth if you are attending a hospital-based scheme. If all goes well and there is no significant haemorrhage at the time of birth—and it is likely that there won't be—you will be able to go home again within 24 hours of giving birth, having had a safe and satisfactory birth experience.

In countries with well-developed home birth services there is a high rate of transfer to hospital because of complications that develop either during antenatal care or during labour. One of the frequent reasons for transfer during labour, especially first labours, is a requirement for pain relief more effective than can be safely given in the home—usually this means an epidural.

In practice, in Ireland transfer to hospital-based care occurs in 40 per cent of pregnancies. While this figure might appear high, it is a similar percentage to other countries that have well-run home birth programmes. In the Netherlands for example, the transfer rate is 45 per cent. One of the most frequent reasons for transfer in labour is because the mother wishes to have an epidural as the labour is more painful than expected.

Reasons for transfer from home to hospital-based care

Conditions developing during pregnancy: diabetes, significant anaemia, haemorrhage, high blood pressure, multiple pregnancy (twins), breech presenation, placenta previa, group B streptococcus and abnormality or death of the foetus

Labour is 14 days or more overdue

Conditions developing during labour: mother's request for epidural for pain relief, haemorrhage, high blood pressure, fever, foetal distress, abnormal presentation (breech, face, brow), slow progress, meconium in the fluid

After delivery if the placenta does not deliver within an hour, if there is excessive bleeding or if you need extra stitching.

Alison (31) had two little girls in London hospitals without any complications and was sent home within 24 hours of having them as is the norm there. She felt strongly that she would want to get back home as soon as possible after her third child was born here.

June Try to find out about Domino scheme. Only women without any previous difficulties or medical problems allowed on scheme. Proximity to Holles Street also important consideration.

July First visits to midwives excellent. Talk through symptoms of pregnancy; given plenty of time and appointments prompt. Blood and urine tested.

August Midwife concerned because I'm so exhausted and am not exercising. She gives me info on swimming and posts more info on yoga. Referred to psychiatrist to talk about post-natal depression experienced with last baby. Excellent experience; he gives lots of good advice about breastfeeding and managing things once the baby is born. Have an episode of bleeding and go straight into hospital to be checked out. Seen very quickly by doctor who confirms all's well with a scan.

September Routine scan at 20 weeks—no waiting and staff give me loads of time—20 minutes at least—

While the previous list may seem intimidating, in practice most of the complications are unlikely to occur and, on a second or subsequent birth, your chances of having a successful home birth are high.

Home birth choices

If you decide on a home birth you have essentially two choices: one is to attend a midwife attached to a maternity hospital scheme and the other is to attend an independent midwife. At the time of writing there are only a few hospital-affiliated home birth programmes. The National Maternity Hospital at Holles Street in Dublin was the first such programme and it is still in operation. If you are interested in home birth you should enquire at your local maternity unit.

Holles Street programme

The Holles Street programme functions in a similar way to other internationally recognised schemes, such as in the Netherlands, which has one of the oldest and most respected programmes in Western Europe. The same team of midwives will look after you throughout the pregnancy. Visits will take place in your home. Your only trip to hospital will be for blood tests and an ultrasound scan. When labour starts two midwives will come to your home and stay with you until after the birth of your baby. In the following days you will be visited every day by your midwife, who will do your baby's heel prick test and advise you about early vaccinations.

Most babies are born on or a few days around their expected date of delivery (EDD). The most precise estimations are based on the results of an ultrasound scan. Even armed with this valuable information, some women who are eager to rush things are tempted to tell people that their due date is earlier than it really is, especially if it falls at the beginning of a month. Doing so won't make the pregnancy seem any shorter—in fact, more often than not, it's more likely to make it seem longer because even if the baby is born on its due date, it will seem 'overdue'. You are better advised to tell people your exact due date, or indeed a couple of weeks later. This will make it less likely that you will be pestered by phone calls from friends and relatives asking 'any news?'.

talking through the scan and explaining different views.

October See consultant who wants to know why I'm interested in the scheme. Reminds me I'll be leaving the hospital as soon as possible after the birth (that's why I'm interested in the scheme!). Next appointment will be with my GP (who can also do my 6 week check).

Mid-January Visit delivery room with midwife. Ooh, very harsh lighting, lots of machines. Bed looks like point of worship or sacrifice, not

exactly homely. Small shower cubicle but no bath. On the personal front, have excruciating pelvic pain in symphysis pubis. Midwife promises to have someone call me.

End January Did yoga class and pregnancy swim class. Teacher urges us to do pelvic floor exercises religiously or pay the price. Advice taken. A few days later, I lean down to pick something up and pain returns and worsens to the point that I can barely move by the weekend. Call midwives first thing Monday

morning (why did I wait?). Appointment made with physio who has to take me upstairs in an ancient lift. Leave with enormous Sumo velcro support belt and exercises to do—transverse abdominals, pelvic floor and buttocks. Physio has explained that labour could be worse or make things completely better. Also advised not to exercise for 10 days and to sleep in some very awkward positions. To make matters worse, varicose veins are popping up all over my body.

Independent midwife

If you decide to choose an independent midwife you may get a recommendation from friends or family, or you may wish to contact An Bord Altranais, which is the regulatory body for midwives in Ireland. In any event you should make sure that your midwife has the backup of a hospital in case there are complications and that she is fully accredited and insured.

You should be completely comfortable with your midwife and confident that should a problem arise you will be transferred to hospital in a timely fashion. One of the problems with childbirth is that emergencies can arise very quickly and sometimes unpredictably. While these situations are rare, you might not forgive yourself if something avoidable were to happen, particularly to your baby, because medical facilities were unavailable.

Domino and early discharge schemes

A good compromise between hospital and home birth is the Domino system, 'domiciliary in and out' which may be in operation in your area. Many doctors who are uncomfortable with the safety aspects of home birth are enthusiastic advocates of this scheme. With Domino your first antenatal visit is in the hospital but all your subsequent visits are in your own home (domiciliary) or a local health centre clinic. Any ultrasound scans or complications are dealt with at the hospital. The

birth plans

There are many elaborate templates for birth plans but by the time you arrive at the hospital you will have tackled a lot of the issues in them already, such as where you are having the baby and who is coming with you.

What you are taught in antenatal classes at your hospital represents the 'birth plan' for that hospital. It is based on vast experience so be wary of plans obtained from other sources. Also be wary of birth plans obtained from sources not in daily contact with delivering women.

Start February See GP and relate how things are starting to improve. Next visit with carers from midwife at home. She spends an hour and takes blood. Monthly appointments go smoothly through March.

End March Attend birth preparation classes with husband. Group of 6 concentrate on labour for 2nd and 3rd time mothers. Last weekly appointments very reassuring, focussing as much on mental state as physical. Advised that with symphysis pubis problem, an epidural is not recommended and that the best delivery position is standing or on all fours.

April Have had a few days of strong Braxton Hicks and attack of diarrhoea. Ring midwives who say that's quite normal and that they expect to see me in the next 48 hours. When labour does start, call and am told to stay home until contractions 5 minutes apart. Stay cool and calm. Go to Holles Street for a check—1 cm and am given option of going back home. Go home, take a bath and suddenly find myself transfixed by the colours of a submersible Winnie the Pooh. Time to go back. Can barely speak and meet midwife whose presence is immediately soothing. Survive on gas and air. Midwife doesn't check how dilated I am but assures me it will be very soon. She knows her stuff and little girl emerges quickly. Floods of emotions, placenta delivered naturally, all over by 5 a.m. At 8 a.m. I'm ready to go home and have breakfast with my older daughters. Visited regularly by midwives all week and delighted to be home.

birth takes place in the hospital (that's the 'in' bit) and all being well, you are discharged home again a few hours after the birth (that's the 'out' bit).

After you have gone home you will receive regular visits from the midwifery team that cared for you during pregnancy. If any significant problems arise during your pregnancy your care will be transferred to the hospital. The Domino system is a very good way to avail yourself of the benefits of continuity of midwifery care. You are looked after by a team you know and who are available 24 hours a day, while at the same time having the back-up of full hospital services if a problem should arise at any stage. The home visits after the birth are also of tremendous benefit. The scheme is not widely available in Ireland at the time of writing so if the concept appeals to you, make enquiries locally through your family doctor or directly to the maternity hospitals.

Another compromise scheme is early discharge home, where birth takes place in hospital but you go home earlier than usual, within 24 hours, and have visits at home for five days in the same way as those who deliver under the Domino scheme.

There is clearly a variety of choices open to you if you do not wish for full-time hospital-based care, shared with your GP or not. The choice is yours, but remember you are making it not just for yourself.

Frequently asked question

Is a birth plan necessary and when should I discuss it with my doctor?

A birth plan (a written wish list for how you envisage your labour and delivery happening in an ideal world) is occasionally helpful but save it until closer to delivery by which time you will have learned a lot more about pregnancy in general—some time after 32 weeks.

If you have a birth plan that differs from your hospital's birth plan make sure to discuss it with your doctor or midwife in good time before your due date. Some hospitals are refusing birth plans because of bad experiences with a minority of women who have caused major difficulties and obstructed staff in their efforts to provide good care, sometimes with poor outcomes for the babies.

It is unnecessary to stipulate things like you don't want to have stitches (no one in their right mind does) or what kinds of intervention are acceptable to you. Presumably, if intervention is necessary you will do whatever you and your medical team determine is best for you and your baby in the circumstances, not what's written down on a piece of paper. Including phrases like 'I would like my baby handled gently', is unnecessary and potentially insulting to hospital staff. Your caregivers are on your side and do their best to make your birth as safe and satisfying as possible.

Your midwife will guide you through the various options during your labour regardless of whether you have a birth plan or not—don't feel you need to have something prepared beforehand.

In summary, a birth plan is not necessary!

what's normal?

Average weight of newborns: 3.5 kg

Less than 2.5 kg: 5.2 per cent

Twins: 2 per cent of all births

Single mothers: 32 per cent

Average age, all mothers: 31 years

Average age, single mothers: 27 years

Home births: 176 (out of 72,000)

Caesareans: 28 per cent

Exclusively breastfeeding: 47 per cent

Non-Irish: 27 per cent

Source: Perinatal Statistics Report 2011
Health Research and Information Division
ESRI (June 2013)

3 antenatal care

The primary purpose of antenatal care is to ensure that all preventable problems are recognised and dealt with as soon as possible. The best care also provides a forum in which advice can be given and questions asked.

You should aim to see your GP, obstetrician or clinic within the first three months of your last period, especially on your first pregnancy. If you have had problems in the past you may wish to make contact earlier or if you have had several uncomplicated pregnancies you may wish to defer your first visit until slightly later. At the first visit your doctor will work out your expected date of delivery (EDD), take a full medical history and carry out a physical examination. Blood tests will also be organised. Antenatal visits are usually scheduled every 4 to 6 weeks up to 28 weeks, every 2 to 3 weeks up to 37 weeks and weekly thereafter. Visits on a first pregnancy tend to be arranged more frequently than on subsequent pregnancies. At each visit your urine will be tested, blood pressure taken and the growth of your baby will be assessed. Ultrasound and other tests will be scheduled from time to time.

start the clock

While conception usually occurs in the middle of the menstrual cycle, the duration of pregnancy is recorded from the first day of the last menstrual period (LMP), some two weeks before. The normal duration of pregnancy is between 38 and 42 weeks. The average pregnancy lasts 40 weeks or 280 days from the LMP. First pregnancies are more likely than subsequent ones to go more than a week overdue.

Expected date of delivery

Your doctor will ask for the date of the first day of your last menstrual period, in order to calculate your EDD—expected date of delivery. He or she will need to know if your cycle is regular and whether or not you recently stopped using the pill, as both may affect your EDD. For example, if you have a 35-day cycle instead of a 28-day one, your due date is probably one week later than average, since ovulation probably occurred on day 21 rather than day 14 of your cycle. Use the chart opposite to work out your own EDD.

Light bleeding after conception

Sometimes a period may not be completely suppressed following conception. You may experience light bleeding or spotting and worry that you are having a miscarriage. An ultrasound scan from six weeks on can help clarify that your pregnancy is continuing if you are in doubt. If you have an early scan and a normal sized embryo is seen, with a heartbeat, the likelihood of miscarriage is very small. There is no point in requesting a scan before six weeks have passed as it will not show enough at this early stage. Even at six weeks the information from a scan may not be conclusive and you may be asked to return in a week or two for a repeat scan.

Even if you experience spotting, you may well continue to have a perfectly normal pregnancy. Any blood lost is from you and not the foetus.

A small proportion of women may also experience episodes of spotting intermittently throughout the early weeks—again with no ill effect on the foetus. This can be frightening but seldom means anything is amiss. However, bleeding may cause some confusion when it comes to calculating the baby's due date until an ultrasound scan is performed. An ultrasound scan from 6 weeks on will help clarify that your pregnancy is continuing.

when is your baby due?

Use the following table to work out your expected date of delivery (EDD). Find the first date of your last period in the bold months, and then just read off the appropriate EDD immediately below. So if your last period started on 25 January, your EDD would be 1 November.

January	1	2	3	4	5	6	7	8	9	10	11	12	13	14	15	16	17	18	19	20	21	22	23	24	25	26	27	28	29	30	31
Oct/Nov	8	9	10	11	12	13	14	15	16	17	18	19	20	21	22	23	24	25	26	27	28	29	30	31	1	2	3	4	5	6	7
February	1	2	3	4	5	6	7	8	9	10	11	12	13	14	15	16	17	18	19	20	21	22	23	24	25	26	27	28			
Nov/Dec	8	9	10	11	12	13	14	15	16	17	18	19	20	21	22	23	24	25	26	27	28	29	30	1	2	3	4	5			
March	1	2	3	4	5	6	7	8	9	10	11	12	13	14	15	16	17	18	19	20	21	22	23	24	25	26	27	28	29	30	31
Dec/Jan	6	7	8	9	10	11	12	13	14	15	16	17	18	19	20	21	22	23	24	25	26	27	28	29	30	31	1	2	3	4	5
April	1	2	3	4	5	6	7	8	9	10	11	12	13	14	15	16	17	18	19	20	21	22	23	24	25	26	27	28	29	30	
Jan/Feb	6	7	8	9	10	11	12	13	14	15	16	17	18	19	20	21	22	23	24	25	26	27	28	29	30	31	1	2	3	4	
May	1	2	3	4	5	6	7	8	9	10	11	12	13	14	15	16	17	18	19	20	21	22	23	24	25	26	27	28	29	30	31
Feb/Mar	5	6	7	8	9	10	11	12	13	14	15	16	17	18	19	20	21	22	23	24	25	26	27	28	1	2	3	4	5	6	7
June	1	2	3	4	5	6	7	8	9	10	11	12	13	14	15	16	17	18	19	20	21	22	23	24	25	26	27	28	29	30	
Mar/Apr	8	9	10	11	12	13	14	15	16	17	18	19	20	21	22	23	24	25	26	27	28	29	30	31	1	2	3	4	5	6	
July	1	2	3	4	5	6	7	8	9	10	11	12	13	14	15	16	17	18	19	20	21	22	23	24	25	26	27	28	29	30	31
Apr/May	7	8	9	10	11	12	13	14	15	16	17	18	19	20	21	22	23	24	25	26	27	28	29	30	1	2	3	4	5	6	7
August	1	2	3	4	5	6	7	8	9	10	11	12	13	14	15	16	17	18	19	20	21	22	23	24	25	26	27	28	29	30	31
May/Jun	8	9	10	11	12	13	14	15	16	17	18	19	20	21	22	23	24	25	26	27	28	29	30	31	1	2	3	4	5	6	7
Sept	1	2	3	4	5	6	7	8	9	10	11	12	13	14	15	16	17	18	19	20	21	22	23	24	25	26	27	28	29	30	
Jun/Jul	8	9	10	11	12	13	14	15	16	17	18	19	20	21	22	23	24	25	26	27	28	29	30	1	2	3	4	5	6	7	
October	1	2	3	4	5	6	7	8	9	10	11	12	13	14	15	16	17	18	19	20	21	22	23	24	25	26	27	28	29	30	31
Jul/Aug	8	9	10	11	12	13	14	15	16	17	18	19	20	21	22	23	24	25	26	27	28	29	30	31	1	2	3	4	5	6	7
Nov	1	2	3	4	5	6	7	8	9	10	11	12	13	14	15	16	17	18	19	20	21	22	23	24	25	26	27	28	29	30	
Aug/Sep	8	9	10	11	12	13	14	15	16	17	18	19	20	21	22	23	24	25	26	27	28	29	30	31	1	2	3	4	5	6	7	
Dec	1	2	3	4	5	6	7	8	9	10	11	12	13	14	15	16	17	18	19	20	21	22	23	24	25	26	27	28	29	30	31
Sep/Oct	7	8	9	10	11	12	13	14	15	16	17	18	19	20	21	22	23	24	25	26	27	28	29	30	1	2	3	4	5	6	7

Medical history

Previous miscarriages

A history of previous miscarriage may prompt your doctor to suggest an early ultrasound scan for your reassurance to confirm that the embryo is developing. If you have had an abortion (termination) in the past, you can be assured that it should have no ill effect whatsoever on your current pregnancy unless there were serious complications like infection or puncture of the womb.

Family history

You will be asked about any family history of diabetes or other inherited conditions in the immediate family. A family history of twins, while interesting, is rarely of major relevance as most women will have an ultrasound scan at some point in their pregnancy that will exclude or confirm multiple pregnancy.

Gynaecological history

A previous history of infertility will be of interest to your doctor as it could influence your pregnancy care. Pregnancies that occur following assisted fertility treatments like IVF may be handled slightly differently. For example, it is unlikely such a pregnancy would be allowed to go significantly overdue. Other events in your gynaecological history are also relevant. Previous pelvic surgery may have resulted in the formation of adhesions, which could cause abdominal pain during pregnancy because they stretch under pressure from the growing uterus. A previous vaginal repair operation or surgery on the cervix for a pre-cancerous lesion (cone biopsy or LLETZ) may have an important bearing on your care during labour and may result in caesarean delivery. A cone biopsy may cause scarring of the cervix so that it does not dilate in labour. Alternatively, treatment for a pre-cancerous lesion may weaken the cervix and result in premature labour. Awareness of previous infectious disease is also important, particularly at the time of delivery. An active herpes blister may necessitate a caesarean section, just as a history of Group B streptococcal infection will require antibiotic treatment in labour.

Medical conditions and surgical history

It is important to tell your doctor about ongoing medical conditions such as diabetes, asthma, epilepsy or high blood pressure and any associated medications, and also to be aware of drug allergies,

antenatal classes

You should make every effort to attend antenatal classes, especially on your first pregnancy. Most hospitals provide classes free of charge and you are legally entitled to time off from work to attend. Night classes may also be available but you may have to pay for these. If you attend classes unconnected with the hospital where you are going to give birth make sure that you go to your place of delivery at least for the classes dealing with labour. This is because hospitals' care plans for labour vary and you need to be aware of the situation in your chosen place. For example, some hospitals will not administer an epidural at less than 4 cm dilation while others are happy to give it earlier. At the classes you will get advice on exercise, diet, what will happen during pregnancy and, of course, the birth itself. The classes provide a great forum for discussion; you will also meet other mothers and learn that your experiences are shared. There is usually a refresher class available for those on second or later pregnancies.

particularly to antibiotics. Previous surgery may influence your pregnancy and how it is managed. Previous surgery to your back, for example, may prevent you from having an epidural in labour.

Lifestyle

You will be asked whether or not you smoke (you shouldn't) and about your alcohol consumption. Ideally, you should avoid alcohol during pregnancy as it crosses the placenta into your baby. In other words, if you have a gin and tonic, so does your baby. There is no evidence, however, that a limited amount of alcohol will cause harm. It appears that alcohol consumption must be considerable and continue throughout pregnancy to cause major problems.

It is not unusual to have drunk a lot in early pregnancy and for it to have no effect on your baby whatsoever. Around Christmas, for example, you might have been at parties and had a lot to drink before you even realised you were pregnant. Don't worry, the chances of damage are tiny.

Physical examination

At your first visit, you may have a general physical examination. You will be weighed so that a baseline figure may be established (if you are significantly overweight this will provide an excellent opportunity to discuss diet and may lead to a referral to a dietician for more detailed advice). You will also be tested for diabetes later in the pregnancy if you are significantly overweight.

Urine sample

At this and every visit thereafter, a sample of urine will be tested for the presence of protein and sugar. Protein in the urine in early pregnancy may suggest a urinary tract infection and sugar may suggest the possibility of early diabetes. Protein in the urine in later pregnancy may be associated with the development of pre-eclampsia or toxaemia. Your urine sample can be from any time of the day and does not have to be kept in a sterile container, although the container should be clean. A small sample is sufficient, about the amount an empty film container or medicine phial would hold.

Internal examination

Sometimes an internal vaginal examination may be performed although generally speaking, it is not necessary, may be uncomfortable and in most cases, contributes no useful information. In some countries, including France and Germany, a vaginal examination is performed at every visit but there is no demonstrable benefit from this custom. In some countries, a cervical smear is also taken at the first visit although it is not standard practice to do so in Ireland.

---

weight

Some caregivers will weigh you at each antenatal visit, but others regard this as unnecessary since if your diet is healthy any weight you gain is pregnancy-related and will go in the few months after delivery. An undue emphasis on weight gain in pregnancy is considered by some to distract attention from the importance of assessing foetal growth.

3D Scans

Many private scanning units offer a 3D picture and video of your scan.

They add nothing to your care. Some couples find the 3D image a little disturbing--almost like an alien!

pre-eclampsia or toxaemia

occurs only in pregnancy, in between 5 and 10 per cent of mothers, mostly first-time mothers. It is a potentially dangerous form of high blood pressure. Signs include excessive weight gain and protein in the urine as well as high blood pressure, and in severe cases, blurred vision, headaches, irritability and acute abdominal pain.

Seizure, or convulsion (eclampsia) is the most serious complication.

The need to detect pre-eclampsia at an early stage is one of the reasons why attending antenatal care and having routine blood pressure and urine tests is so important.

If you have a mild case, you will be kept under observation as either an out- or inpatient and labour will be induced as soon as the cervix ripens. If the disease progresses, you will be given medication to prevent convulsions and your baby will be delivered immediately.

Abdomen check

The doctor will check your abdomen for any swelling or scars. In the first three months of pregnancy, the abdominal examination usually will not reveal any swelling as the uterus can normally only be felt rising out of the pelvis after week 12 at earliest although on a second or subsequent pregnancy it may be felt earlier. If the uterus is felt to be larger than expected, the pregnancy may be further advanced than thought or you could be expecting twins. There may be some other reason such as a fibroid or ovarian cyst but this is uncommon. If there is a significant difference between the actual and expected size of your uterus, an ultrasound scan will clarify the issue. If the uterus is significantly smaller than expected, it may mean that the pregnancy is not as advanced as was thought. A smaller than expected uterus is unlikely to indicate a problem like miscarriage, particularly in overweight women, unless there has been accompanying bleeding or a rapid disappearance of pregnancy symptoms. Again, if there is concern, an ultrasound scan will clarify matters.

Breast examination

A breast examination is primarily intended to exclude lumps. Other minor deviations from normal, such as inverted nipples or small skin tags on the nipple are of no consequence. They do not prevent breast-feeding and do not require any treatment. Many doctors are of the opinion that breast examination is unnecessary as it is extremely rare to find anything out of the ordinary.

Blood pressure

It would be unusual for your blood pressure to be elevated in the early stages of pregnancy but it will be checked at every antenatal visit to confirm that it is staying within normal limits. High blood pressure (hypertension) is usually not accompanied by any other symptoms. Headache, particularly in early pregnancy, is rarely a symptom of high blood pressure. Headache in early pregnancy is not at all unusual and can often by cured by a paracetamol tablet, which is harmless to your baby.

Blood pressure readings are noted in two figures: the systolic (higher reading) and diastolic (lower reading). Normal values are anything below 140 systolic and 90 diastolic. It is normal for blood pressure to dip very low in pregnancy and readings of 90/60 or less are not uncommon. Low blood pressure may make you feel faint or dizzy from time to time. This is not harmful to your baby.

Don't be worried if you are told your blood pressure is low. This is normal in pregnancy and far better than having it high.

Heart check

In Western societies today it is very unusual to detect heart disease for the first time during pregnancy. Because blood flow increases so dramatically during pregnancy, benign murmurs in the heart are not unusual, however. If you have a history of rheumatic fever as a child you may have some residual valve damage, which might cause a strain during pregnancy. This is unusual nowadays and most heart conditions in pregnant women are the result of congenital problems present from birth and have almost always been recognised prior to pregnancy. Most will have been treated surgically and present no problems during pregnancy.

Blood tests

Blood tests will also be organised and may include the following screenings:

Blood group

This is important to know, especially if you are rhesus negative and the father of your baby is rhesus positive. Fifteen per cent of the Irish population is rhesus negative. Problems as a result of different blood groupings are rare but may cause serious problems for the baby. If you are rhesus negative you will probably be offered a protective dose of anti D at approximately 28 weeks. This is to prevent you from developing antibodies to your baby's blood.

Haemoglobin

This measures your blood iron level and will determine when, or if, you need supplemental iron. If your periods have been very heavy before pregnancy, your iron level may well be reduced. A low haemoglobin level (anaemia) presents no risk to the baby but may accentuate the fatigue characteristic of early pregnancy.

Rubella immunity

This tests your resistance to German measles, or rubella. If you have been immunised in the past or had rubella yourself, you are likely to be immune. If you are not immune, you need to avoid contact with children who have the infection because it may damage your developing baby. Again, in modern Western society it is unusual, though not rare, not to have immunity to German measles.

checks and tests

Each antenatal visit includes a check on a urine sample for protein (infection or toxaemia in later pregnancy) and glucose (possible diabetic tendency); a blood pressure measurement and an examination of the growth of your baby. Later in pregnancy, particularly the last 4 weeks, the position of your baby in the womb becomes more important—if it is breech (bottom first) for example, it will probably result in a caesarean birth.

welcome advice?

Once you have told people about your pregnancy, or your pregnancy begins to show, prepare to be on the receiving end of all sorts of unsolicited advice—sometimes from perfect strangers. It may be difficult to distinguish between good advice and utter nonsense. As a general rule, ignore advice to avoid certain activities like lifting, stretching, active sports and sex—pregnancy is not an illness and your developing baby is well protected in the womb. If you are in doubt about any aspect of your pregnancy, ask your doctor or midwife—don't rely on hearsay.

WR test

This refers to the Wasserman test for syphilis, which is performed routinely in most societies. A positive result is rare and may be falsely positive due to a condition that produces antibodies that interact with the WR test. Syphilis is tested for because it is treatable during pregnancy and failure to treat it may cause damage to the baby.

HIV

This is the test for antibodies to the virus that causes AIDS, and is done on a routine basis. HIV is a difficult virus to contract unless your behaviour has been 'high risk' in the past. High-risk behaviour includes intravenous drug abuse, promiscuous sex or unprotected sex with a partner in a high-risk category. HIV is more common in certain communities—in Central Africa, for example—and amongst bi-sexuals. If a woman is HIV positive, there is a risk of transmitting the virus to the baby but this risk can be reduced dramatically by treatment during pregnancy.

Hepatitis

You may be screened to see if you are carrying the hepatitis virus, of which there are several types. The most common is hepatitis B. It is important to know if someone is positive for two reasons: firstly, the baby will require treatment after birth to prevent infection (which is 95 per cent effective) and secondly, because the pregnant woman may unwittingly infect her caregivers and/or partner. Hepatitis C is less common but presents the same risks. Hepatitis may be contracted via contaminated blood products, sex with a carrier or intravenous drug abuse.

Toxoplasmosis

Although most countries do not test routinely for this disease (except France), it is common for women to show evidence of past exposure to it (20–30 per cent in New York, 90 per cent in Paris). Past exposure, during which antibodies will have developed, protects against further infection. In other words, if you've had toxoplasmosis you won't get it again. The infection is acquired by eating undercooked meat or by coming in contact with cat faeces—it is therefore very avoidable by taking simple precautions. Cook meats well and be very careful when handling cats. Always make sure you wash your hands well before eating.

Chickenpox

Many hospitals will now perform routine testing for immunity to chickenpox (varicella). If you have had chickenpox in the past you, and your baby, are fully protected. Shingles arises in people who have had chickenpox in the past. It is not infectious.

Ultrasound

Ultrasound is very widely used in modern obstetrics and it is unusual not to have at least one routine scan during your pregnancy. It will provide you with your first-ever look at your baby inside you and for most women, the first scan is a landmark event, complete with a photo opportunity. While most scans are not necessary from a medical point of view, ultrasound has become an integral part of antenatal care and most doctors recommend at least one scan in the first half of pregnancy. There is no evidence that ultrasound harms the foetus in any way.

The best time to have a scan is between 18 and 22 weeks because this is when the most information can be gleaned from it, including the due date and whether the baby is a boy or a girl. In some clinics, a scan may be performed at your first visit, even as early as six weeks, but the information gained then is limited to confirmation of a heartbeat and estimation of dates.

If there is a need to test for the risk of Down syndrome you may be offered a scan earlier than usual to confirm dates before having the tests.

When having a scan you lie on a hospital bed with your head and body propped up semi-upright. The ultrasonographer puts a transparent gel on your abdomen. This helps the handheld part of the scanner (which is a bit like a computer mouse) to glide easily over your skin. If you have a cameraphone you may wish to take a photo/video of your scan, but do ask the ultrasonographer first. High frequency sound waves, which cannot be heard by the human ear, are then bounced off the uterus and its contents and are reflected, or echoed, back on to the machine. The reflections build into a black and white image on a video screen. The picture is constantly updated so that foetal movements are clearly visible.

Detecting Down syndrome

Women over 35 tend to be anxious about the possibility of their baby having a chromosomal abnormality—in particular, Down syndrome. It is clear that there is a gradual increase in risk corresponding to advancing maternal age for this condition. Previous obstetric history and family history are irrelevant, except in the rare case of one inherited type of Down syndrome, which can occur at any age. The actual risk for an individual can be estimated by a nuchal thickness scan and blood test at 11–13 weeks.

The nuchal area is at the back of the baby's neck. The result of the scan is available immediately. If the risk is high the question of definitive testing, by either Chorion Villus sampling (CVS) or

detecting abnormalities

Modern ultrasound machines can detect a number of abnormalities or 'markers' for specific conditions, including Down syndrome. These are subtle findings, primarily relating to the thickness of a fold of skin at the back of the neck (nuchal thickness). The presence of these markers indicates a risk rather than a definitive diagnosis, which can only come from chromosome analysis of samples obtained by either amniocentesis or CVS. Not all conditions can be detected by ultrasound.

maternity leave and entitlements

Many women wait as long as possible to tell their employer they are pregnant. While it is important to choose your moment well, (and take your employer's needs into consideration) remember that you have certain unalienable rights as an employee, which are not compromised by your being pregnant. If you have been in your job for more than one year, your employer is legally bound to keep your job for you and must give you 18 weeks' maternity leave plus the option of an additional eight weeks' unpaid leave. While two weeks' leave is supposed to fall before the birth, many women choose to work as long as possible up until the birth and save their leave until afterwards when it can be rolled into whatever holiday time they are due.

However, try to take at least a fortnight off before your due date. You will be more tired at the end of your pregnancy than you may think when you are making your plans for maternity leave.

For more information on maternity leave, contact the Department of Social and Family Affairs—preferably before you make your announcement.

amniocentesis, will be discussed with you. A CVS test involves passing a fine needle into the placenta and aspirating a sample of tissue for genetic testing. The result of the test is usually available in two weeks, although there is a test which only takes three days—QFPCR (see A–Z). It is not widely available in Ireland. An amniocentesis is usually performed later than a CVS and involves passing a fine needle into the fluid surrounding the baby, withdrawing a sample and doing a similar genetic analysis. Both procedures, CVS and amniocentesis, have an inherent risk of miscarriage of approximately 1 in 100.

NIPT, non invasive pre-natal testing

NIPT is a relatively new method of testing for chromosomal abnormalities. It involves taking a blood sample from the mother at any time from 10 weeks onwards. Fetal DNA, known as 'cell free fetal DNA', is in the mother's bloodstream from this stage of pregnancy on. The blood sample is sent to a laboratory outside Ireland, usually to the United States, and analysed there. The conditions that it can help to diagnose are Down syndrome (trisomy 21) Edward's syndrome (trisomy 18) and Patau's syndrome (trisomy 13). Edward's and Patau's syndromes are two very serious conditions which are almost always fatal either before birth or very soon after. The test can also help to diagnose excess numbers of the sex chromosomes, X and Y. There are normally two sex chromosomes present, XX for a girl, and XY for a boy. An extra sex chromosome is rare but can cause significant abnormalities, including intellectual disability and fertility problems in later life, although in most cases the effects are mild and may not be noticeable at all. The test results usually become available in 10 days. In about 3 per cent of cases not enough fetal DNA can be extracted to give a result and the test may need to be repeated. The test can be performed in donor egg IVF pregnancies if there is only one fetus, and in twin pregnancies conceived either naturally or by IVF with the mother's own eggs. The result will be expressed in terms of 'very low risk' , 'less than 1 in 10,000' or 'high risk'. It is very reassuring if you get a low risk result. However, to get a definitive answer you will still need to have either an amniocentesis or chorion villus sample (CVS) test. The NIPT test is not available on the health service and you will have to pay for it; the cost is about €700, including a scan to date the pregnancy accurately.

Is it a boy or a girl?

The best time for visualising the baby's sex is after 24 weeks, although it may be possible for the scanner to see it at 16 weeks. In general, predictions are 80–90 per cent accurate. It is becoming increasingly common for women to ask if the scanner can tell what sex their child is and in Ireland, scanners will do their best to see if asked. Most hospitals are reluctant to do a scan solely to determine the baby's sex because this consumes resources that are better directed towards women with problems.

Frequently asked questions

How soon can I tell if I'm pregnant?
The first day after your period is due although some women suspect, correctly, that they are pregnant much earlier. If you are pregnant most over the counter tests will register positive even before you miss your period.

How can I get the most out of my antenatal visits?
Be informed—read this book! Learn about pregnancy in general and keep a list of any queries you may want the doctor or midwife to answer at your next appointment.

When should I start antenatal classes?
At your first visit you will be advised about antenatal classes, which should be booked early. They are a fantastic learning tool and a great place to meet other mothers and fathers who will be as eager to discuss different aspects of pregnancy and birth as you are. Most hospitals offer an introductory class followed by a series of classes later on.

Are iron supplements necessary?
Not unless your haemoglobin tests indicate your iron levels are low. If in doubt a check on your iron levels during pregnancy will clarify matters.

Is there such a thing as a stupid question?
There is, of course, but that shouldn't stop you asking! Especially in a first pregnancy you cannot be expected to know what is normal and what is not.

I am 36, I've just found out I'm pregnant and I'm worried about the risks. What are they?
There is a slightly increased risk of early miscarriage. There is an increased risk of chromosomal abnormality with advancing age. The risk is 1 in 950 or 0.1 per cent at age 30, 1 in 350 or 0.28 per cent at 35 and 1 in 100 or 1 per cent at 40. The most common chromosomal abnormality is Down syndrome, or trisomy 21. Other, less common, chromosomal abnormalities include trisomy 18 (Edward's syndrome) and trisomy 13 (Patau's syndrome)—both are usually fatal soon after birth. There is no increased risk of structural abnormalities like spina bifida or cleft palate. You can be tested for these abnormalities early in your pregnancy if you wish.

4 general health in pregnancy

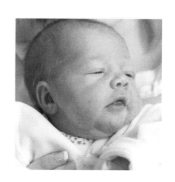

Luckily, most women are healthy when they get pregnant and remain so throughout pregnancy. Unless you suffer from a pre-existing condition such as diabetes, or you develop a complication like high blood pressure, there is no reason why pregnancy should affect your health in anything but a positive way. Pregnancy presents an opportunity to focus on your diet and living habits with the intention of improving your general health. It's a time to look after yourself, not just the growing baby inside you. Listen to your body and common sense.

Diet

At the beginning of pregnancy, you may feel nauseated and perhaps suffer from vomiting, but these symptoms usually recede after 12–14 weeks at the latest. Your diet may suffer as a result, but there's no need to worry—your baby is getting adequate nutrition. Food is passed across the developing placenta through the bloodstream in a very basic, molecular form as carbohydrate, protein, fat, vitamins and other essential nutrients to the baby. Your own body has adequate stores to keep the embryo well fed at this early stage of pregnancy. Remember, the embryo only weighs about 40 grams (1½ ounces) at 12 weeks so needs very little in spite of growing at a phenomenal rate.

If you don't eat well, it is most unlikely that the child will be deprived of any nutrients essential for growth and development because your body tissues will be broken down in order to supply your baby with adequate nutrition. In other words, if you are found to have low iron levels, it is you who will suffer until they are corrected rather than your baby.

As a general rule, bear in mind that you are establishing eating patterns for life and the earlier you put an emphasis on a balanced diet, the better everyone's health will be.

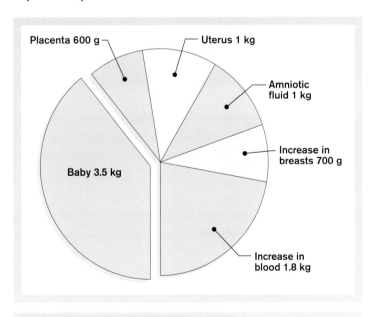

WHAT WEIGHS WHAT (AVERAGE) AT TERM
Remember, these are approximate figures only. There are lots of perfectly normal variations from the average.

morning sickness

So-called morning sickness and fatigue are legendary millstones of early pregnancy—but they are by no means universal. Many women sail through early pregnancy without the slightest bother. Still others find the emotional shock of imminent parenthood more dramatic than any physical symptoms. Whatever the case, pregnancy is a tremendous learning experience and a physical adventure.

Folic acid

Folic acid with multivitamins is the only dietary supplement doctors recommend. It should be taken as early in pregnancy as possible (ideally for the three months prior to conception) because folic acid supplementation is directed specifically at preventing neural tube defects such as spina bifida, hydrocephaly and anencephaly. The embryo's spinal cord will already have closed by the end of the fourth week of pregnancy so early supplementation is best. If you do not start taking supplementation early on, do not be overly concerned—chances are that if you eat a healthy diet, you already take in enough nutrients from it.

Folic acid is also thought to protect against other abnormalities including cleft lip and palate. Apart from folic supplementation, you need not worry about your diet from the baby's point of view. If you eat well, both you and your child will have access to all the important vitamins and minerals.

increase in blood volume

Within weeks of conception, a pregnant woman's blood volume increases by approximately 40 per cent—an extra 1.2 litres. This massive increase, combined with the muscle relaxing effects of the pregnancy hormones, accounts for the headaches you may experience in the first three months of pregnancy.

Iron

Iron supplementation is usually unnecessary, although it used to be recommended to everyone. Unless your diet is deficient in iron (something to watch if you're a vegetarian) or you are showing signs of significant iron deficiency, you don't need it and it is also blamed for indigestion or constipation. High iron intake may decrease the risk of your baby developing eczema and asthma. Fatigue, particularly in early pregnancy, is rarely a sign of anaemia. If you are prescribed iron, it will turn your stools a dark brown or black. It is usually easier to take iron in tablet form, with food, to avoid stomach upset.

calorie values

Recommended daily calorie intake during pregnancy: approximately 2,600 in total—an extra 500 calories per day.

Remember that not all calories are created equal. 210 calories from a packet of crisps are not as beneficial to you as 210 calories from a fresh fish fillet or dressed salad.

Weight gain

It is not unusual to gain a few pounds in early pregnancy but some women may worry that if their early rate of weight gain continues they will put on a huge amount of weight. This need not be a cause for concern. Nor should failure to gain weight. Many women actually lose weight in the first three months due to nausea and/or sudden aversions to particular foods. Weight loss is rarely associated with a problem in the baby and makes it easier to re-establish pre-pregnancy weight after delivery.

Weight gain varies enormously from one woman to the next and normally bears no relation to the baby's size. The average woman gains between 10 and 15 kg (20–30 lb) over her pregnancy. If you gain more than this, it will be difficult for you to lose the extra weight but if you stick to a sensible, well-balanced diet, take a reasonable amount of exercise and avoid fatty foods, any weight you gain will be accounted for by pregnancy and will be lost after it is over.

If you eat junk food you will put on weight whether you are pregnant or not. Only you can control your diet and only you will really know what you are eating.

From the very beginning of your pregnancy, keep a gentle eye on the weighing scales so that a significant gain or loss can be noted but don't worry about maintaining your weight gain at a constant level. It will fluctuate. Heavier women may find they gain less weight initially, or even overall. Don't worry about not putting on weight as long as your baby is growing at a normal rate which will be confirmed at antenatal visits. If you are concerned in any way, consult your doctor.

Cravings

Cravings have no scientific explanation as yet but they are thought to reflect the body's need for certain minerals and vitamins. There is no reason not to indulge them as long as the target foods are not unreasonably high in calories and fat and low in nutritional value. Go ahead—have a pickle with your ice cream. Just don't have the whole container. Some cravings are quite bizarre, for example, petrol fumes! Try to be sensible in your response to any cravings you may develop and if in doubt ask your doctor. It's also normal not to have any cravings.

Constipation

The muscle relaxing effect of pregnancy hormones on the bowel can cause constipation and bloating. If you are taking iron tablets you may blame them when in fact it's your hormones that are to blame. Before trying a prescription, make some healthy adjustments to your diet. Drink more fluids and eat more bran and fibre—perhaps mix muesli or bran into your morning cereal, choose a grainy brown bread rather than processed white or grab a fruit for a snack. Check the nutrition information on various foods for fibre content and try to ensure that you are eating at least 18 g of fibre per day (easily accomplished). A serving of baked beans (13 g) plus five tablespoons of bran flakes (5 g) would do the job for a day.

good sources of important nutrients

Protein: Meat, fish, eggs, dairy products, peas, pulses, beans

Vitamin D and calcium: Dairy products, tinned fish, green vegetables, bread. Vitamin D is made in your body by exposure to sunlight, so being out of doors every day is helpful. Most breakfast cereals are fortified with both Vitamin D and calcium (as well as folic acid and iron).

Iron: Beef, potatoes, legumes, soy products, molasses. A fall in your haemoglobin, or iron level, is normal in pregnancy because of your increased blood supply, which dilutes the iron that is already present in your blood.

Folic acid: Green, leafy vegetables are your best bet although many commercial cereals and breads have folic acid added to them.

Golden rules

- Make dietary adjustments as soon as possible so that you feel healthier.
- Vary your diet to include a wide variety of proteins, vitamins and minerals.
- Minimise your intake of sugar, salt, butter and fatty foods in general.
- Avoid alcohol, undercooked or raw meats and fish with high mercury contents (shark, tuna, king mackerel).
- Don't drink too much tea or coffee: the caffeine they contain can cause a pregnant woman's heart to race.
- Advice to avoid peanuts is controversial. An increase in peanut allergy among children is more likely to be due to rubbing creams containing peanut-derived oils into babies' skin than to eating peanuts during pregnancy.
- Eat moderate amounts of dairy products, lean meats, fish, nuts, pulses and eggs.
- Do not eat unpasteurised soft cheeses or pâtés because of the small risk of developing listeriosis, an uncommon infection that might cause few, if any, symptoms in a mother but can infect the placenta and then the baby.
- Avoid any food that is in and out of the fridge, including salads, as exposure to warm temperatures encourages the growth of the listeria bug.
- Eat lots of vegetables, fruit, high fibre cereal and breads.

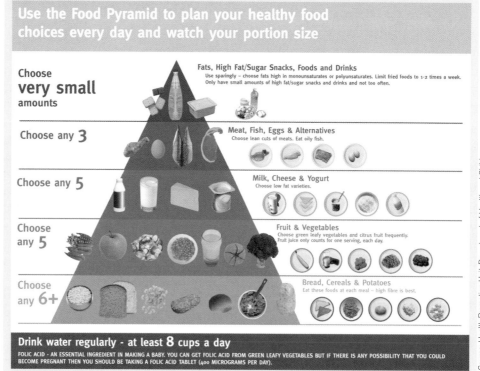

Use the Food Pyramid to plan your healthy food choices every day and watch your portion size

Choose **very small** amounts

Fats, High Fat/Sugar Snacks, Foods and Drinks
Use sparingly – choose fats high in monounsaturates or polyunsaturates. Limit fried foods to 1-2 times a week. Only have small amounts of high fat/sugar snacks and drinks and not too often.

Choose any **3**

Meat, Fish, Eggs & Alternatives
Choose lean cuts of meats. Eat oily fish.

Choose any **5**

Milk, Cheese & Yogurt
Choose low fat varieties.

Choose any **5**

Fruit & Vegetables
Choose green leafy vegetables and citrus fruit frequently. Fruit juice only counts for one serving, each day.

Choose any **6+**

Bread, Cereals & Potatoes
Eat these foods at each meal – high fibre is best.

Drink water regularly - at least 8 cups a day
FOLIC ACID - AN ESSENTIAL INGREDIENT IN MAKING A BABY. YOU CAN GET FOLIC ACID FROM GREEN LEAFY VEGETABLES BUT IF THERE IS ANY POSSIBILITY THAT YOU COULD BECOME PREGNANT THEN YOU SHOULD BE TAKING A FOLIC ACID TABLET (400 MICROGRAMS PER DAY).

Source: Health Promotion Unit, Department of Health and Children

Alcohol

Moderate amounts of alcohol taken in pregnancy do not appear to cause any problems to the developing baby. Nevertheless, the best advice is to restrict your intake to a minimum until the lowest 'safe' level has been scientifically determined. There is mounting evidence that while a moderate amount of drink won't harm the baby, it does have an effect. Research has shown that even tiny amounts appear to slow an unborn baby's reflexes in the same way that an adult's reflexes are slowed. As with adults, the effect is transient.

Most women lose their taste for alcohol early in pregnancy anyway—this is probably due to an innate protective mechanism. Despite this, only one-third of all mothers-to-be avoid alcohol completely. If you have consumed what you consider to be an excessive amount of alcohol (enough to give you a hangover), don't worry. It would have been better not to have done so, but there is no evidence that an occasional episode of drinking will harm a developing baby.

Foetal Alcohol Syndrome is only associated with significant and regular alcohol abuse throughout pregnancy and occurs in only a tiny percentage of babies. Babies born with the syndrome fail to grow normally, have specific facial features (mainly involving the eyelids) and brain abnormalities that cause irritability, hyperactivity and sometimes mild mental retardation.

public property

As soon as you are noticeably pregnant, absolute strangers as well as some friends and family will feel compelled to give you unsolicited advice about your pregnancy. It can seem that everyone has a story to tell and everyone's an expert. Take it all with a grain of salt and ask your doctor about any issues that seriously concern you.

Smoking

You should not smoke, actively or passively, when you are pregnant. Smoking is clearly dangerous in the long term for anyone—pregnant or not—but is associated with several serious problems in the foetus. There is a higher rate of miscarriage, failure of the baby to grow properly, death of the baby before birth and premature delivery among women who smoke because smoking reduces the baby's supply of oxygen and nutrients and so impairs its ability to grow properly. There is also a higher rate of sudden infant death syndrome associated with babies born to mothers who smoke. Given these facts, there is absolutely no justification for smoking during pregnancy or in the post-natal period. If you find it impossible to stop completely, at least cut back as much as you can. Choosing a low tar-content cigarette makes no difference. Remember, every time you have a cigarette, so does your baby. You are unlikely to offer a five year old a puff, so why force your unborn child to have one?

Keeping fit

If you exercise regularly when you are not pregnant you should continue to do so while you are—but stick to low-impact aerobic exercise only. Your training target pulse rate should stay below 140 beats per minute. Swimming, walking, cycling, pilates and yoga are best. Swimming is probably best of all—women who swim regularly do tend to have less complicated labours. The weightless feeling of swimming, particularly towards the end of pregnancy, is also especially relaxing, and the breathing control is very helpful in labour. Avoid contact sports like hockey and sports like (water) skiing and riding where there is potential for trauma to both you and the baby. If in doubt, ask for a professional opinion.

During pregnancy, an aptly named hormone, relaxin, is secreted, which loosens all the ligaments that bind the joints together. Its effects are most marked in late pregnancy when the pelvis prepares to expand slightly during labour to facilitate birth. At this stage, women are particularly susceptible to over-extension of the joints, causing undue strain and pain in the lower back, chest and pelvis. Because your ligaments are loose, stretching movements that overextend the joints should be avoided. Golf, for example, serving at tennis and even heavy gardening may aggravate any tendency to lower back pain.

Shortness of breath during exercise is normal during pregnancy. As long as you can breathe comfortably, don't worry. Some women get breathless during even the mildest exercise like going up a flight of stairs in pregnancy—this rarely represents anything serious. If in doubt, ask your doctor. A baby does not suffer from lack of oxygen if you are breathless.

American College of Gynaecology guidelines on exercise during pregnancy

1 Regular exercise (at least three times per week) is preferable to intermittent activity. Competitive activities should be discouraged.

2 Vigorous exercise should not be performed in hot, humid weather or during a period of febrile (feverish) illness.

3 Ballistic movements (jerky, bouncy movements) should be avoided. Exercise should be done on a wooden or tightly carpeted surface to reduce shock and provide sure footing.

4 Deep flexion or extension of joints should be avoided because of connective tissue laxity. Avoid activities that require jumping, jarring motions, or rapid changes in direction.

5 Vigorous exercise should be preceded by a five-minute warm-up. This can include slow walking or stationary cycling with low resistance.

6 Vigorous exercise should be followed by a period of gradually declining activity that includes gentle, stationary stretching. Because

Skin changes

It is normal for your skin to become darker during pregnancy. This may be especially marked around your nipples and also in a line from your belly button to your pubis, the linea nigra. You will also notice that any moles you have will darken. If you are worried about them show them to your doctor. These will fade back to their pre-pregnant colour after delivery.

Some women find that they get spots for the first time since adolescence rather than 'blooming'. This unpleasant development is due to changing hormones. If your skin gets very bad mention it to your doctor before using harsh medicinal creams. Roaccutane and tetracycline should not be used under any circumstances.

Small red spots, which may be itchy, are common in pregnancy and usually go away after delivery. They can occur anywhere on your body but are more common on your trunk or hands. They are called spider naevi because they look like little spiders.

Itchiness, sometimes associated with a rash, can be a problem in pregnancy. Itchiness of the abdomen is common and is due to the skin stretching. It will disappear after pregnancy and has a 50 per cent chance of happening to you again if you get pregnant again.

There is a form of itchiness in pregnancy associated with a slowing of liver function. Your doctor may order a blood test to clarify if this is a problem. In severe cases where there is also jaundice, there may be an increased risk to your baby's health. Your doctor will give you the appropriate treatment for your symptoms—perhaps a light steroid cream or antihistamine tablets—although little appears to work where slowing of liver function is the problem.

gentle exercise

Many gyms and dance studios offer special exercise classes for pregnant women. These usually concentrate on gentle stretching exercises that will keep you limber as you grow. They can also help strengthen sensitive areas like the back. Yoga is especially popular now and is particularly beneficial because the deep breathing techniques it employs are very similar to those recommended in labour. Ask your antenatal class teacher for recommendations or ring gyms near you for more information about classes.

car safety: strap in

Seatbelts are essential during pregnancy. They should be positioned as normal to curtail contact with the steering column of the car in an accident.

connective tissue laxity increases the risk of joint injury, stretches should not be performed at maximum resistance.

7 Heart rate should be measured at peak activity.

8 Care should be taken to rise gradually from the floor to avoid orthostatic hypotension (low blood pressure that occurs on rising to the erect position). Some form of activity with the legs should be continued for a brief period. Begin with activity of very low intensity (walking or marching in place) and advance gradually.

9 Activity should be stopped and a physician consulted if any unusual symptoms appear.

10 Strenuous activity should not exceed 15 minutes in duration.

11 No exercise should be conducted in the supine (lying down) position after the fourth month.

12 Caloric intake should be adequate to meet the extra caloric needs of pregnancy as well as the exercise performed.

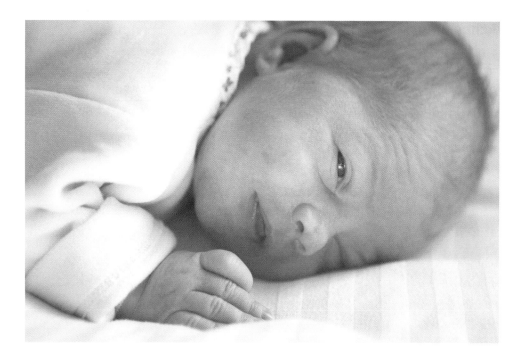

Stretch marks

Stretch marks may develop over your tummy and breasts as they expand, especially in late pregnancy. No treatment with oils or creams has proven effective in getting rid of them, despite many claims to the contrary. Stretch marks do fade after delivery but will never completely disappear. The best offence against them is a good defence—try not to gain too much weight so the skin will not be forced to stretch too much in vulnerable areas.

different each time

If you have already had a child, and are used to being pregnant, it can be difficult to assimilate the fact that each pregnancy is different and needs to be treated individually.

Sex

Your enthusiasm for sexual activity, or libido, may wane during pregnancy. This is particularly true in the early stages when you may feel nauseated and tired or suffer from tender breasts. Some women, however, find the opposite is true. They may relish the changes in their bodies and develop new, or heightened, physical awareness that in turn fuels an increased sex drive. Later in pregnancy, most agree that an expanding uterus can make intercourse a bit awkward, necessitating changes in position. These are normal, temporary developments and partners should be encouraged to be tolerant of them. If both parties are willing, there is no reason why any form of sexual activity should be restricted during pregnancy. Intercourse does not cause miscarriage or premature labour.

Aches and pains

Pregnancy can represent a major physical challenge, which is often expressed as a series of various aches and pains in different parts of your body. Almost every pregnant woman is afflicted by some minor aches and pains at some stage. This is because the pregnancy hormone relaxin relaxes all the ligaments in your body. Your pelvis may be significantly affected because it is made up of several bones bound tightly together by ligaments. When these ligaments relax, bones that normally don't move scrape against each other and this movement can be painful.

At the front of the pelvis is the pubic symphysis joint. If this loosens, as it normally does in pregnancy, the rubbing of the two adjacent pubic bones can produce a pain described as a knife-like stabbing, low down in the front of the pelvis and sometimes in the vagina. Sometimes the joint may loosen up completely so that the bones are completely separate. This is a regular, though uncommon, event known as a spontaneous symphysiotomy or symphysis pubis dysfunction. The hip joints, and particularly the lower back joints, can all be similarly affected and produce a variety of aches and pains in the pelvis, the lower back, hips and sometimes pain down the back of the leg on one or both sides (sciatica). Not everyone gets these aches and pains. If you do develop them they may not be severe and will often pass of their own accord. Do mention them at your next antenatal visit, though, because sometimes physiotherapy can help ease symptoms.

As the baby grows the uterus will push internal organs, mainly bowel, out of the way. This puts pressure on your upper abdomen and rib cage. The rib cage is often stretched and a nerve may get caught under it. This can be quite painful.

Various types of abdominal pain are not unusual during pregnancy. In the early stages, particularly on a first pregnancy, you may get crampy pains as your uterus stretches for the first time. Unless the pain is very severe, or associated with bleeding or a dark discharge, you needn't be worried. Crampy pains in your abdomen are not unusual and unless persistent or severe are rarely significant. Pain on either side of the abdomen low down is not unusual either and is often due to the stretching of ligaments that support the uterus. This type of pain is more common in a first pregnancy because the ligaments are stretching for the first time.

contact your doctor or hospital without delay if:

you have some bleeding after 26 weeks, your baby's movements have decreased dramatically

you have a severe headache and upper tummy pain and are also feeling generally unwell, any time from 24 weeks on

you are genuinely concerned about your own or your baby's health.

let your doctor know at your next visit if:

you have felt weak or dizzy, or have been fainting

you have developed a troublesome ache in your side or back

you heard something about the hospital where you are planning to have your baby that disturbed you

you have been to antenatal classes and don't fully understand some points made there

Take a note of anything you are concerned about so that you will remember to bring it up at next visit.

Heartburn

Heartburn is another of the effects of the muscle-relaxing hormones. The condition is due to a relaxation of a circle of muscle at the lower end of the oesophagus, the tube connecting the mouth to the stomach. This relaxation allows acid to travel from your stomach up into your oesophagus—heartburn! Try eating a little often and don't eat spicy foods. If your symptoms are particularly bad you may be prescribed a tablet that cuts down acid production in your stomach, thereby removing the source of the problem. Over-the-counter antacids are often successful in easing heartburn.

Leg cramps

In pregnancy, the threshold for muscle spasm drops, so you are much more likely to experience cramps, particularly in the calves. Depending on your luck, and level of fitness, it could be that you suffer a bit from jittery legs or you could wake in the night with an agonising cramp so severe you cannot straighten your foot without help. Bad cramps can leave you with a very sore calf for days, which some might even mistake for a suspected blood clot. The fitter you are, the less likely you are to have major cramps. In some cases, taking a calcium supplement suppresses the tendency to cramps. Stretching exercises before bed will not help prevent cramps but a hot water bottle applied to the sore area may give some comfort after it's over.

excruciating cramps

Anne (22), a post grad student in history swam three times a week throughout her pregnancy as she had before she got pregnant. 'I would sometimes get the most excruciating cramps in the arch of my foot when I was kicking in the pool or in my calf at night. They were so bad I couldn't actually straighten my foot out at all and put it flat on the floor. I would yelp with the pain. At night my partner would literally have to pummel where it hurt with his fist and if it was my foot, force it straight. For hours after I could feel the tension and soreness and it felt like it could go again at any minute. I seemed to get them less if I massaged them just before bed.

Fluid retention

Fluid retention may cause swelling of your ankles, particularly in the evening if you are on your feet a lot during the day. Put your feet up or soak them in cold water for relief. Fingers may also swell so that rings become too tight to remove. It may be necessary to have the rings cut off in a jewellery shop. Fluid retention may also cause some stiffness in your joints in the morning. Retaining fluid does not mean you are developing toxemia. Like many inconveniences of pregnancy all you can do is deal with the symptoms rather than avoid or cure the problem. Reducing your salt intake has no effect on fluid retention. Do whatever makes you feel more comfortable.

Carpal tunnel syndrome is also due to fluid retention compressing the nerves as they pass through your wrist into your hand. Symptoms of carpal tunnel syndrome include numbness or tingling in the tips of the fingers and weakness of the hand muscles. Occasionally, symptoms may be so severe as to make it impossible for you to work or hold a cup. Sometimes a splint may help, particularly at night. Fortunately, carpal tunnel syndrome goes away following delivery.

Time off work

You may continue working during pregnancy as long as your work is not overly demanding physically. You should plan on taking at least two weeks off at the end of the pregnancy, more if you are pregnant with twins, in case you feel tired. You will usually be planning when you will stop work at a stage of pregnancy when you have plenty of energy and feel you could keep going forever. As you near term you may find this changes, so build a little flexibility into your plans if you can.

Near term, you may also find your concentration lapses. Many women who work with figures or in front of computers find their minds going blank from time to time. Others find their reaction times slow or discover they have forgotten to do routine things. Don't worry—forgetfulness is a normal phenomenon. If possible, try to keep your work hours flexible and keep an open mind about finishing work earlier than usual if necessary. Working right up until labour is fine from a physical point of view and doesn't harm the baby in any way but is probably unnecessary. You should be able to organise your work so that your colleagues and clients are not suddenly abandoned as a result of something reasonably predictable like imminent birth.

Travel

Travel by air is generally not a problem when you are pregnant, with a few caveats. Don't travel abroad if your pregnancy is in any way complicated. For example, don't travel if the placenta (afterbirth) is lying over the cervix as there is a risk of bleeding. This will have been noted at your 18–22 week scan. As a general rule, you should not fly much beyond 34 weeks, or six weeks before the baby is due. This is because of the risk of premature labour or some other complication occurring out of the blue in a foreign environment, not because travel in itself is dangerous. If something was to go wrong, your travel home could be restricted and you might find yourself spending the last six weeks of pregnancy away from your partner, family and usual medical attendants. Insurance cover varies from company to company but many airlines and holiday operators may not offer satisfactory insurance beyond 28 weeks. Check with your travel agent and/or insurer to verify coverage.

If you are making a long-haul trip at any stage, make sure you drink plenty of water during the flight and walk about frequently as well as doing the aerobic exercises detailed in your in-flight magazine. Flight socks will also help. Pregnancy predisposes to the formation of blood clots and long periods of inactivity along with dehydration further

Mary (25), a solicitor, was determined to stay at her desk until the minute she went into hospital. She was worried that her colleagues in her new office wouldn't approve of her taking time off before the baby was born when she was more or less at the beginning of her career. By the time she was 37 weeks pregnant however, Mary was too tired to put in her regular 10 or 11 hours and found herself flagging. 'Looking back, I don't know what I was trying to prove. No one would have cared if I was gone for the last two or three weeks. After all, they were already planning for me to be gone for a few months anyway and I'm sure my boss, having had three children herself, had contingency plans for cover in place for the last couple of months of my pregnancy in case something went wrong.'

increase the risk. Check with your doctor before planning such a trip. As far as miscarriage is concerned, if you are beyond ten weeks, the chances of it occurring are small no matter where you are and flying certainly doesn't make it more likely.

If you need vaccinations for travel in underdeveloped countries, check with the vaccinator prior to having them. As a rule, dead viruses pose no threat and avoiding a serious disease is far preferable to contracting the disease and having treatment for it. For example, taking a little quinine is far less harmful to a foetus than a full blown case of malaria.

Frequently asked questions

I fly a lot for work. Will the air pressure changes affect my pregnancy?
No. You may retain more water than usual and your feet and ankles may swell considerably but flying will not harm your baby at any stage of pregnancy. See also *Travel* on page 45.

Is spotting after sex normal?
No, but it is very unlikely to represent a problem. You should always tell your doctor about it if it recurs because you may have some minor condition like a polyp, which might need treatment.

I have a history of miscarriage. Should I avoid sex in the first three months?
Sex in the first trimester, and throughout pregnancy, is very safe. There is no evidence that it causes miscarriage.

Is bathing safe?
Yes, but avoid douching.

What should I take when I have a headache?
Take paracetamol, not aspirin, for minor aches and pains but inform your doctor of any chronic ailments.

People have been telling me that I look very big and that I have too much fluid. Should I believe them?
They're probably wrong. Only your doctor or midwife can assess your condition and size although lay people persist in passing personal comments of this nature. It's probably worth mentioning the remarks at your next visit if only to reassure you that there is nothing to worry about.

Is it ok to eat peanuts during pregnancy?
Yes, there is no evidence that eating peanuts during pregnancy has any adverse effect whatsoever on your baby.

5 your pregnancy month by month

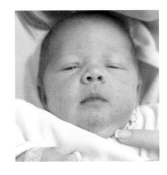

Every month brings milestones in your pregnancy and you are likely to spend a lot of time imagining exactly what is happening to your baby as the days go by. As your pregnancy progresses you will notice many changes in your body. In the early weeks when the pregnancy hormones get going some women find the changes overwhelming, to others they are merely incidental. Some people notice nothing at all. How you feel in early pregnancy has no bearing on your baby's health.

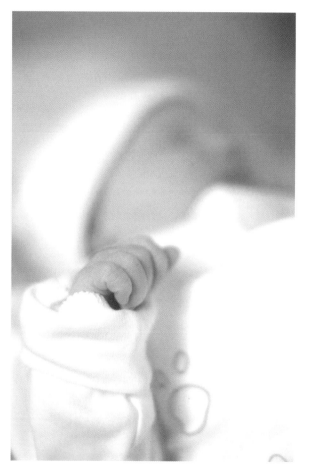

The middle part of pregnancy, from approximately 20 to 28 or 30 weeks, is generally the easiest time. Your energy levels will return to normal and any 'morning' sickness you have suffered from will usually have gone. You will be fairly comfortable because your bump is not too big, your baby is moving in a reassuring way and you can notice its continued growth. Complications are rare during this time and you will only need to visit your doctor or antenatal clinic once a month at most.

In the last three months of pregnancy, you will see your doctor or midwife more frequently. On a first baby, you will have appointments scheduled every two to three weeks after 28 weeks and every week after 37 weeks. This will give you plenty of opportunity to ask questions, as will the antenatal classes you should be attending.

Weeks 0–4

The duration of pregnancy is dated from the first day of your last menstrual period (LMP). This means an embryo is only two weeks old by the time the so-called first four weeks of pregnancy have passed and you are about to miss your first period. Indeed, you may not even realise you are pregnant during the first four weeks of pregnancy. Symptoms that might suggest you are pregnant include a more frequent need to empty the bladder, a slight tingling feeling in the breasts and perhaps, an unusual metallic taste in the mouth. You may also find you go off certain foods and alcohol. It is also perfectly normal to notice nothing different at all. A home pregnancy test will resolve any doubts. Home tests should turn positive within two weeks of conception, possibly before you have even missed a period. The test reacts to the presence of a pregnancy hormone, HCG (Human Chorionic Gonadotrophin), in your urine and is most concentrated in your first sample of the day.

The developing embryo consists of a ball of cells, hollow in the middle, called the blastocyst. The blastocyst implants into the prepared wall of the uterus approximately 8–14 days after conception, then burrows in and begins to develop further. Meanwhile, the ovary starts to produce more progesterone and this prevents menstruation.

urination

Frequency of urination is a common feature of early pregnancy because of the rapid increase in circulating blood volume as well as the pressure of the enlarging uterus on the bladder. This symptom usually subsides after the first 8 to 10 weeks. It may return again in the latter stages of pregnancy when the weight of the baby puts sustained pressure on your bladder.

Weeks 5–9

A small number of women notice no changes whatsoever in their bodies at this stage but, during the second month, full pregnancy symptoms, which most women will be aware of, usually develop. You may have some crampy pain in your pelvis due to your uterus stretching, particularly in a first pregnancy. Rapidly increasing hormone levels, particularly of progesterone, will affect many different parts of your body. Progesterone has the effect of relaxing all the muscles in your body, including those in your bowel. This causes the feeling of lassitude, often compared with jet lag, which can last for the first 18 to 20 weeks of pregnancy. You may find yourself fit for nothing but sleep in the evening. Many women find taking naps and going to bed much earlier than usual irresistible in early pregnancy—particularly if they have other young children. Listen to your body and give it the rest it's asking for. It's all too easy to overextend yourself and get run down if you don't. If pregnancy has not been confirmed, this lack of energy may be mistakenly attributed to anaemia.

Breast enlargement, sometimes dramatic, can be noticeable as early as six weeks. Breast tenderness usually accompanies the change in size as the milk-producing glands develop. The tenderness usually abates within the first three months of pregnancy although a sensation of fullness persists. Some women are alarmed by how much and how soon

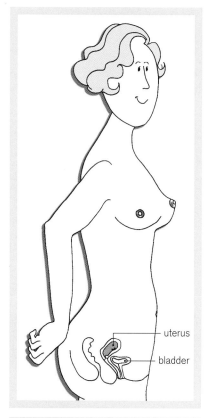

uterus

bladder

6–8 WEEKS
The 6-8 week old foetus already has a rudimentary brain, a closed spinal cord and a primitive heart whose beats may show on a scan. At 8 weeks arm and leg buds have grown and the foetus is about 2.5 cm (1 inch) long. You won't notice any change in your own shape just yet. Note how close your bladder is to your expanding uterus. As your baby grows there will be increasing pressure on your bladder and you will find yourself urinating more frequently.

their breasts grow and need to be reassured that they will not keep growing at a constant rate throughout the pregnancy. A properly fitted 'nursing' bra will provide the necessary extra support and some relief from discomfort.

You will probably need to urinate more often due to your increased blood volume—initially your kidneys will respond to this by trying to expel more urine.

Nausea, and possibly vomiting, may become pronounced. Because of this, or for no apparent reason, you may find yourself giving up certain foods and alcohol or craving unusual foods. Try to avoid junk foods and chocolate so you don't gain too much weight at this stage or get more nauseated. You may feel bloated and constipation may also cause you discomfort.

The presence or absence of any of these symptoms will make no difference to the health of the embryo growing inside you. There is no good explanation as to why some women experience almost no symptoms of pregnancy and others are completely floored! The health of your developing baby is unrelated to how you are feeling.

The embryo grows and develops tremendously in the first eight weeks of pregnancy. By the end of the sixth week, the spinal cord has closed, a rudimentary brain has formed and a primitive heart is beating, which may be seen on an ultrasound scan. Tiny limbs begin to develop and by the end of week eight, arm and leg buds are present. Eyes, ears and other facial features are beginning to form but have not yet taken on a fully human appearance. The foetus, which is almost doubling in size every week during this period, measures approximately 2.5 cm (1 inch) in length.

Now is the time to consider what form of antenatal care you would like and where you wish to deliver (see Chapter 2).

nausea
It is normal to have some degree of nausea and/or vomiting in the first eight to ten weeks of pregnancy. As long as some liquid or food is staying down there is no cause for concern. If nothing is staying down then you will be admitted to hospital for re-hydration and intravenous fluids. Although it is unpleasant, excessive vomiting that requires admission to hospital (hyperemesis) does not harm the developing foetus in any way whatsoever.

Weeks 10–14

You may continue to feel tired but any nausea and breast tenderness will usually begin to ease by week 12. The pressure of your swelling uterus on your bladder may still cause greater frequency of urination but should not be confused with a urinary tract infection. Your doctor may feel your uterus rising out of the pelvis depending on its position and how heavy you are. At 12 weeks, the risk of miscarriage is less than 5 per cent, so many women choose to tell others about their pregnancy now. Your first antenatal visit should be scheduled between weeks 10–12.

The third month of pregnancy is a time of rapid growth for both foetus and placenta. Attached to the placenta by its umbilical cord, the foetus floats in the amniotic sac like an astronaut in space. The amniotic sac provides plenty of room for it to move around and exercise developing limbs. The foetus begins to drink the amniotic fluid and its kidneys start to produce urine, which is passed back into the amniotic sac. After birth, urine contains waste products from the body's metabolism, but before birth, elimination of waste is taken care of by the placenta, so foetal urine is simply clear, clean water. The placenta also performs several other major functions of the body. In the uterus your baby is effectively in an intensive care unit. It is on a kidney dialysis machine, a ventilator for its lungs, and is being fed intravenously—all functions performed by the placenta! An incredibly sophisticated and versatile organ, it also produces hormones.

At the end of week 12, the foetus has two arms and legs, the ovaries or testes have formed (although it is too early to see them on a scan) and it measures approximately 5 cm (2 inches) long. Movement is clearly visible during a scan. The placenta develops by week 12 to the point where it takes over the production of progesterone from the ovary. The foetus weighs about 40 g (1½ oz).

Weeks 15–19

As your waistline swells, pregnancy becomes increasingly obvious. A dark line, the linea nigra, may form between your belly button and pubis. Likewise, your nipples will begin to darken and surface veins on the breasts may become more pronounced and bluish.

Nausea is probably due to the pregnancy hormone HCG (Human Chorionic Gonadotrophin). It can make you feel sick at any time, day or night (not just in the morning). You will probably stop feeling ill by week 12 but in a minority of cases, some feeling of nausea persists throughout pregnancy or returns in late pregnancy. The presence or absence of nausea and/or vomiting has no bearing on the pregnancy itself.

Pronounced nausea is sometimes associated with twins, but not always.

The best way to curb nausea is to eat a bland diet, free of 'challenging' foods such as curries and hot, spicy foods as well as high-fat food like deep-fried chips. It may also help to eat small amounts frequently rather than the usual three square meals.

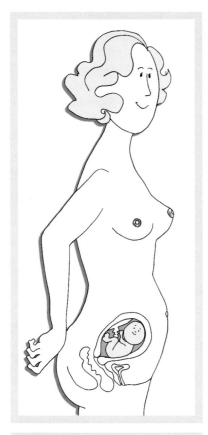

19–20 WEEKS
The foetus is now about 19 cm (8 inches) long and weighs about 350 g (12 oz). All the organs have been formed, arms, legs, fingers and toes can be seen. Your bump will probably start to show.

gaining weight

The rate of weight gain varies greatly although around half a kilogram (one pound) a week is average for the middle three months and the period of most weight gain is from 20 to 30 weeks.

Depending on your build, you may still be able to hide a growing bump behind loose fitting clothes. You may notice growth surges in your uterus, literally overnight. It is not unusual to feel foetal movement around week 18, although in a first pregnancy you may not notice it until 22 weeks. Heavier women tend to notice the movement, or so called quickening, later than slim women while women who have already had children may notice it as early as 15 weeks. Many women describe the initial sensation as feeling like bubbles bursting in the stomach, or fluttering. Up to 26 weeks, it is not at all unusual to go for a day or two without noticing movements, even if you have felt them before. This is particularly true if you are busy and preoccupied with other events in your life. A placenta situated on the anterior, or front, uterine wall may also mask foetal movements by acting as a buffer between the foetus and the abdominal wall.

Growth and development continue during these weeks so that by the end of week 19 the foetus measures approximately 19 cm (8 inches) long and weighs approximately 350 g (¾ lb). The ears and eyes are developing rapidly and the foetus can hear sounds outside the uterus. Many mothers notice foetal reactions to loud music or sounds; the foetus meanwhile begins to recognise the mother's voice as distinct from others at the end of this period. The foetus' sense of touch and also fingernails are well-developed at this stage. A fine downy hair, lanugo, covers the body. The lungs are not yet sufficiently developed to support life outside the womb but by week 16 the foetus is more or less completely formed. The remainder of pregnancy is taken up by growth and subtle developments in the various organs. At this stage, it is very unusual for the foetus to die or for premature delivery to be necessary. However, the foetus has no hope of survival if delivered now.

Weeks 20–24

By week 20 you are halfway through your pregnancy and you will probably find that your energy levels improve and any residual nausea disappears. Symptoms due to the expanding uterus become more noticeable now. 'Growing' pains, particularly in a first pregnancy, can cause discomfort low on each side of the abdomen. The uterus pushes the bowel out of the way as it expands so you may begin to experience a feeling of fullness after eating only small amounts. Heartburn, or acid indigestion, may worsen from this time onwards as your stomach moves up towards the lower oesophagus (the tube from your throat to your stomach). Progesterone, the muscle-relaxing hormone, has loosened the band of muscle separating your stomach from your oesophagus.

It is unlikely that you will be able to continue wearing your normal clothes after this point.

Your breathing may also become a little more laboured and noticeable due to the expanding uterus putting pressure on your diaphragm. Pregnancy hormones will also make you breathe more deeply so that you blow off more carbon dioxide than when you are not pregnant. You will probably gain about 500 g (1 lb) per week during this part of pregnancy. Ignore comments about how small or large your bump looks because no one can possibly know how your baby is growing just by looking at you.

24 weeks represents the lower limit of viability, or the time at which survival outside the womb is a possibility. In fact, very few babies survive if born this soon. Their organ systems still need further development. The baby's lungs develop to the stage where they are capable of exchanging oxygen and carbon dioxide, although considerable further development is necessary for them to function normally on their own. The baby's sense of touch and hearing become more sophisticated and movements become smoother and less jerky in nature. By 24 weeks, the baby weighs approximately 500 g (1¼ lb).

when am I really due?

It is important to clarify your due date in the first half of pregnancy —when the most accurate predictions can be made from a scan—so that you'll know when and if you go past your due date. If your scan doesn't fit your own dates by 10 days or more, the scan date will be regarded as more accurate. If the scan gives a different date it doesn't necessarily mean you've miscalculated, it just means you conceived in a different part of your cycle.

Weeks 25–29

The rapid growth of the baby will accentuate all of your existing symptoms. Heartburn, for example, may become more frequent, your breathing more noticeable and your bladder more sensitive. Your breasts may also start to produce and leak colostrum, a

Braxton Hicks' contractions

At any time from 28 weeks onwards you may feel your uterus harden with mild contractions. These are not labour pains and are known as Braxton Hicks' contractions. They don't occur in every pregnancy but are a normal, common feature of late pregnancy. They are different from labour pains because they are not painful and do not intensify in strength as they progress. Some women even say they feel quite nice. They may be sufficiently strong to make you stop what you are doing for a few seconds but they are much shorter and more sporadic than true labour contractions, which build and come at closer intervals without relenting.

You will be able to sleep through a Braxton Hicks contraction but a real labour pain will definitely wake you. Likewise, a series of Braxton Hicks' contractions may last a few minutes and then stop for a few hours or days, whereas labour contractions will not stop and start for long periods.

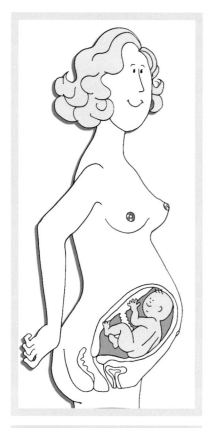

32 WEEKS
Your baby now weighs about 2000 g (4 lb). He or she can hear sounds outside the uterus and also, now that the eyelids are open, responds to light. If born now, your baby has a very good chance of survival. You will be less comfortable now, with various aches and pains.

sweet, watery, yellow-tinted fluid full of vital nutrients that will give the baby sustenance before your milk comes in. This leakage is perfectly normal, even if it does not happen to everyone and has no implications for your ability to feed your baby. There is nothing you can do to stop it happening. If you are planning to breastfeed, it is not necessary to take any special care of the breasts at this stage—manipulation will not make feeding easier. In the past it was sometimes recommended to try to express pre-milk or colostrum to facilitate breastfeeding but this is of no benefit. You may find that a drop or two of colostrum stains your underclothes every now and then and want to invest in disposable breast pads early on.

If you have not already been fitted for a pregnancy bra, you should do so now (even if you have, you may find it no longer fits by the end of your pregnancy). Good support will help keep you from straining your back and may give a great deal of comfort. Some women find that it is more comfortable to sleep in a bra towards the end of pregnancy, too.

You may find it difficult to get comfortable in bed and low back pain may start to become a problem, particularly if you lead a very sedentary lifestyle. Minor aches and pains in the abdomen, back and chest are all typical from this stage on.

In these four weeks, the baby will at least double in size, so that it weighs approximately 1.2 kg (3 lb) and measures 28 cm (11 inches) by week 29. Foetal movements become much more noticeable and at your week 28 antenatal visit, it will probably be possible to determine in which direction the baby is lying, head-down being the most common. If your baby is not head-down at this stage, don't worry. There is plenty of time for it to turn. The baby's eyelids are now open and responsive to light. With modern neonatal intensive care, the chances of your baby surviving premature birth are very good from week 26 on.

Weeks 30–34

During this month you will probably have one or two antenatal visits, with particular emphasis on checking your blood pressure and urine to detect pre-eclampsia (toxemia), and to confirm that your baby's rate of growth and alignment in the uterus are normal. Usually, the baby will line up with its head down (cephalic presentation) from now on but in some pregnancies, particularly second or subsequent pregnancies, the baby may not settle into its final position until much later. The increasing weight of the baby will place a strain on your lower back. You may also find that you are getting unusual pains in your pelvis as the ligaments binding your joints together loosen in preparation for labour and delivery. Waking at night from cramps in your feet and legs and a need to empty your bladder are not at all unusual.

Foetal movements become stronger and may even be vigorous enough to wake you at night. They may cause pain if the baby kicks you in the rib cage. Most often, however, they feel pleasant—like a localised, if sporadic, massage. Very vigorous movements do not indicate distress —a baby lacking in oxygen actually slows down its movements to conserve energy. If you do not feel movements constantly, don't be concerned as long as you feel ten in a day. These may all occur at the same time, perhaps ten kicks in a row.

If you are concerned that movement has diminished, count each movement to reassure yourself—hiccups are considered individual movements and are a good sign that the baby is healthy. Foetal hiccups are recognisable as a pulse-like regular movement. They may last for more than an hour. Some women may not notice them at all, don't worry if you don't. If you are concerned about how much your baby is moving, go to the hospital where staff can check the baby's heart rate with an electronic tracing or ultrasound. Babies do not go completely quiet prior to labour starting but the character of their movements does change in the lead-up to birth. Movements become more squirmy and involve less kicking when space is at a premium but the baby should still be making ten movements a day. Movements are often most noticeable at night time when you yourself are resting and not distracted by your daily activities.

By week 32 the baby weighs approximately 2 kg (4 lb) and the head is in proportion to the body. If born prematurely the baby would have an excellent chance of survival although some assistance with breathing and feeding would be needed as well as some time in a special care baby unit.

antenatal classes
are best started around week 30, which gives you plenty of time to complete a full course of classes and discuss all aspects of your impending birth with other mothers and experts. These classes will have particular significance for first-time mothers and their partners. The classes will lay out the hospital's birth plan. As this will be based on years of practical experience, you should be wary of plans taken from books or the Internet that are often based on scanty evidence or personal experience.

hiccups
The baby practises breathing which is jerky, like hiccups. These are a very healthy sign, but not every mother with a healthy baby will notice them.

Weeks 35–39

You are likely to become increasingly awkward as the baby and you put on more and more weight. You may notice more aches and pains in your lower or upper back, or in the pelvis. Carrying a late pregnancy is as cumbersome as carrying a full rucksack 24 hours a day—with the added disadvantage that the baby may like to squirm and kick when you want to sleep and is indiscriminate in where she or he aims those kicks!

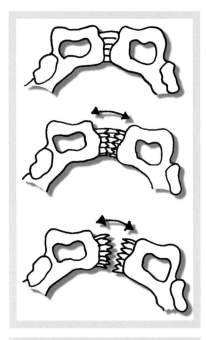

PUBIC SYMPHYSIS JOINT

The pubic bones are joined by tendons (like the Achilles tendon in your heel). During pregnancy, these tendons may relax so that the two bones rub together, causing pain. The tendons tighten up again after delivery. Sometimes the tendons tear and the two bones separate completely; this is known as a spontaneous symphysiotomy. The tendons will heal again without intervention.

Heartburn may become a problem in the latter half of pregnancy as the baby gets bigger and pushes up against your stomach. For mild heartburn, simple remedies—antacids and small, bland meals, will help. Fatty foods like chips and spicy foods like curries will cause most women in their last few weeks of pregnancy considerable discomfort. Antacids available in chemists pose no harm to the baby—in fact, most are calcium-enriched, which is a plus. Sleeping slightly upright may also help keep unpleasant things down. Heartburn may ease once the baby's head 'drops' or enters the pelvis to become engaged. This usually happens around week 36 in first pregnancies but may not happen until right before birth in subsequent ones. The fact that your baby's head has engaged does not mean that labour is going to start soon. The head can engage at 34 weeks and labour not start until 41 weeks or the head may not engage until the day before labour starts. The head tends to engage earlier in first pregnancies.

Your pelvis will also loosen considerably from now on. Some women notice a sharp stabbing pain in the vagina on occasions. This is a result of a slight separation of the pubic symphysis, the point at the very bottom of your abdomen where the two pubic bones are joined together and is a normal physiological event in preparation for labour. You will probably find it increasingly difficult to get a good night's sleep. If you have a birth plan that differs from your hospital's birth plan, you may want to go over it with your doctor at one of your weekly antenatal visits.

Most women feel tired and forgetful towards the end of pregnancy so allow for two weeks off work preceding the birth if you can and rest as much as possible. Many women find it difficult to sleep in the latter part of pregnancy. For some, it is because they can't get comfortable, for others it is because they have to empty their bladders several times

the baby's positions

Don't worry about the position of your baby's head before or during labour. By week 36 your baby has a greater than 95 per cent chance of being in the right position—that is head down. If your baby is breech, or bottom first, you will probably be advised to attend your doctor to see if the baby can be turned to a headfirst position. This is usually done at 37 weeks and is known as an external cephalic version (ECV). If you have had several children your uterus is more stretchy and so your baby may not settle into its final position until closer to delivery.

If your baby is changing position constantly this is known as an 'unstable lie'. You may be advised to come into hospital from 38 weeks because of the risk of either your waters breaking or labour starting during the night. Many find their minds racing. You may find yourself physically tired but mentally wide awake. Many women also have the most bizarre dreams imaginable towards the end of pregnancy and these can be quite disturbing and disruptive. If you are getting exhausted, discuss the problem with your doctor. Sleeping tablets for one or two nights may help to break a cycle of sleep deprivation and associated mental stress. The last thing you want is to go into labour when you are worn out for lack of rest. There will be plenty of sleepless nights ahead!

You may find your concentration slipping towards the end of pregnancy and this is completely normal. Many women comment that they lose their way while driving familiar routes, fail to remember to stop at stop signs or become forgetful. You may find yourself losing your train of thought in the middle of a conversation or a discussion at work. This kind of memory lapse is typical of late pregnancy.

Breathlessness is very common towards the end of pregnancy, partly because of the extra weight you are carrying and partly because the diaphragm is pushed up by the expanding uterus. Slow down and try to regain control with nice, even breaths if you are puffed. If the breathlessness is very severe, mention it to your doctor. Shortness of breath does not mean your baby is not getting enough oxygen. The only condition where a baby may not get enough oxygen from its mother is a rare form of heart disease that virtually immobilises the mother. Bad attacks of asthma or pneumonia, for example, do not result in any danger to your baby.

Stress incontinence, or leakage of urine when coughing or laughing is also very common in late pregnancy but should go away after the baby is born. Some women may think their waters have broken. If your waters go you will have a sudden gush and continue to be wet or dribble fluid afterwards. If it occurs close to term you will probably

time off work

Ideally, you should try and take the last two weeks preceding the birth off from work. Use this time to relax and nest—prepare the baby's room and the rest of the house (stock the cupboards, etc.) and tend to loose ends. Some people are superstitious about getting things ready for a baby until after the birth; if you feel this way, turn your attention to other things. Indulge in lunches with friends, a trip to the cinema, a nap—whatever treats you can— because time will be at a premium soon enough. While you don't want to strain yourself, it's a good idea to keep busy enough so that the time doesn't pass too slowly. The countdown is on but the last few weeks can seem like an eternity, especially if you go overdue.

with your baby lying across your womb. This risk is very small because a baby will usually stabilise as the uterine muscle tone improves with the beginning of labour. There is also an equally small risk of cord prolapse if your waters go. If your baby stays as either a breech or unstable lie,

the likelihood of your having a caesarean section increases significantly. There is no proven way that you can manipulate your baby into the proper position yourself.

The position of your baby's head is of no relevance whatsoever until labour starts. During labour your

baby's head will normally rotate so that its face is pointing to your back. If the head rotates so the face is facing your tummy (occipito-posterior position) this may have no effect on your labour, may slow the labour, or in rare circumstances you may need a caesarean section.

get contractions soon after, within a matter of hours. Leakage of urine tends to be intermittent. It can be confusing and if you are in real doubt, check with your doctor or hospital. Pelvic floor exercises tend not to be terribly effective in preventing stress incontinence before birth, although they are very helpful in strengthening the area after birth so that the problem does not persist in subsequent pregnancies.

The baby's internal organs continue to mature, its hearing further improves and it moves more purposefully in the womb, although space is very limited due to its size. The character of the activity changes from kicking and vigorous, sharp movements to more twisting, pushing and turning types of movement as the baby gets bigger and has less room to manoeuvre. By week 35 most babies have settled into a head-down position. If your baby is breech (bottom-down) at this stage, your obstetrician or midwife may suggest trying to turn it right way round (external cephalic version) at 37 weeks. If this is not successful a caesarean delivery is highly likely.

The baby's lungs produce a substance called surfactant, which prevents them from collapsing after birth. Thumb sucking is common. The placenta continues to transport nutrients and oxygen and remove waste. The baby continues to drink amniotic fluid, passing increasing volumes of foetal urine and meconium, or solid waste, from the bowel. Male babies' testicles will have descended into the scrotum. By week 39, the average baby weighs just under 3.2 kg (7 lb) and measures approximately 50 cm (20 inches).

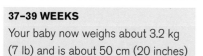

37–39 WEEKS
Your baby now weighs about 3.2 kg (7 lb) and is about 50 cm (20 inches) long.

Weeks 40–42

During the last four weeks of pregnancy, your mind will naturally focus on the impending birth. If the pregnancy continues past the EDD (and half of all pregnancies do), anticipation may give way to grumpiness. If this is your first pregnancy, you will naturally be apprehensive about the prospect of delivery and may well wish it were all over.

One way to look at labour and delivery at this stage is to remember that it will take no more than several hours in total, while the actual delivery of your baby itself will be over in a matter of minutes. As an exercise, look at your watch now; go back twelve hours and see what you were doing; now come forward again to the present moment—if your labour had started twelve hours ago there is a better than 90 per cent chance that you would be sitting in bed holding your newborn baby! In fact, the average length of time a first labour takes, from the time of arrival in the labour ward to delivery, is less than seven hours in the National Maternity Hospital, Holles Street. It is even shorter, by approximately half, in subsequent labours. The better your understanding of the actual process of childbirth, the more confident you will feel. Before your antenatal classes end, try to learn as much as possible about the various types of pain relief available—the respective advantages and disadvantages—so you can make an informed decision about what course to take during labour before the big day. Keep an open mind, however, particularly on your first birth, as you cannot possibly know what it is going to be like for you as an individual.

The average baby gains weight at the rate of 1 per cent per day from weeks 36–40 so that it weighs approximately 3.5 kg (7.5 lb) on average at full term. Most of its lanugo (downy body hair) has disappeared although many babies are born with downy shoulders, arms, legs and foreheads. This hair falls out after birth. True to legend, all babies are born with blue eyes although the colour may change within minutes of birth. Vernix, a waxy substance, is particularly thick around the neck and skin creases but the amount of it present at birth decreases in babies born after their due date.

If you are overdue

Your due date falls 40 weeks after your last menstrual period. Most women go into labour within a few days either side of their due date. However, with a first baby, it is not at all unusual to go a week to 10 days past your due date. Obviously, the longer you go over, the more likely it is you'll become anxious and fed up and start thinking about induction. In general, your best chance at having a normal labour and birth is if you go into labour yourself without being induced.

Frequently asked questions

I'm ten days overdue and fed up. Is there any truth in any of the old wives' tales about ways to start labour?
Nothing you can do will help start labour. Do not try taking castor oil, which will only give you stomach cramps (and possibly diarrhoea) as opposed to contractions. Sex will not trigger labour either although there is prostaglandin in sperm. Neither will a long walk!

the last two weeks

Deirdre (36), a writer and mother of three, now remembers the last two weeks of her last pregnancy with a shudder. Although her first two children were born more or less on time, her last went 12 days over.

'If one more person rang up and started their conversation with 'are you still there?' I was going to scream . . . and then kill them. It was bad enough sitting around waiting without everyone else watching the kettle boil, too. But when my doctor finally made a date to induce me I felt ambivalent. I'd heard that induction was more painful and it just didn't fit into my mental picture of what I thought the birth was going to be like based on the other two. I really wanted to get on with it and had asked to be induced so I was surprised at my reaction. The night before I was supposed to be brought in I went into labour myself and it was such a relief. It was like my body was reacting to a deadline.'

I want to breastfeed. Is there anything special I should do in late pregnancy to facilitate it?
No. Expressing colostrum, the yellow fluid secreted by the breasts before milk comes in and massaging the areolae and nipples prior to birth will not make feeding easier once the baby is born.

I am about to have my second baby and its head is engaged. Does this mean I'm likely to go into labour soon?
No, but it makes it less likely that you will go overdue.

I'd like to know which part of my bump is which part of the baby. Any tips?
It is extremely difficult, even for medical students, to tell what's what by feel. Chances are that the baby's bottom is at the top of your abdomen. You may also feel or even be able to see feet or elbows pressing against your skin when the baby tries to adjust its position or moves in late pregnancy.

Is it OK to sleep on my back?
Yes. In theory the weight of a pregnant uterus can compress major blood vessels supplying the uterus. In practice, this doesn't appear to happen while you sleep. Your body will respond by moving and changing position. You may get dizzy if you lie on your back while awake and that is a sign to move. Videos of people sleeping show that most people move around a lot in their sleep so even if you start off on your back and end up on your back, chances are you will have moved around in between.

I'm 26 weeks pregnant with my second child and I can barely walk (which was never a problem before)—the baby seems to be so low. Is there anything I can do to alleviate the pressure, especially as things are only going to get worse.
Your symptoms are not unusual in a second pregnancy. Many mothers say they feel the baby is going to fall out, so pronounced is the pressure. Don't worry, your baby is not going to fall out! These symptoms are due to stretching of your pelvic supports, which have lost a significant amount of their elasticity as a result of your first pregnancy. This is one of the reasons why a second birth is usually so much easier, and quicker, than a first. The only way to make matters easier is first of all to recognise that these symptoms are to be expected, and secondly try to adapt your activities to find more comfortable positions. The good news is that these sensations do not represent anything sinister and they will go away after your delivery.

The doctor suggests I should have a sweep at term. What is a 'sweep'?
A sweep refers to an examination of your cervix where a finger is inserted into the cervix and swept in a circular fashion. The idea is to bring on labour. It is at best uncomfortable, sometimes painful, may cause bleeding and is only moderately successful. I do not recommend it.

6 labour and delivery

Labour is the process by which normal birth takes place. If you are healthy there is no reason why you should not be successful in achieving a normal birth after a normal labour. Some women have a fear of childbirth that relates to a lack of confidence about their ability to give birth, often not helped by lurid tales of disaster from friends. Everyone's birth experience is unique to them, so don't apply others' experiences to yourself. You and your baby are unique individuals and although there are common threads in labour that are almost universally applicable, your birth is special to you—both of you!

In addition to the medical care you receive, your personal pain threshold and your psychological ability to cope with both the pain and the intensity of the experience as a whole will ultimately determine how you perceive the experience of labour. If you are well informed about what labour entails and the various options open to you, you will be better able to shape the course of events to your liking. Birth can be exciting and exhilarating; a positive and pleasant experience is within every woman's grasp.

is this a pregnancy or a labour pain?

You may have episodes of quite strong contractions and wonder if labour has started.

Labour pains are so strong they stop you in your tracks and will wake you if you are asleep; they are regular and your whole abdomen becomes very hard and tense.

Pregnancy pains are shorter, are often sharp, and are not accompanied by regular hardening of your whole abdomen. You may have pain around, or under your belly button or at the top of your tummy in the centre—this is not unusual.

When does labour start?

On average labour starts 9 months, or 280 days, following the first day of the last menstrual period, or 266 days following conception. No one is sure why, or how, it starts.

Since conception can occur at a varying time during the cycle there is a range of dates when labour is likely to start. From your own point of view, however, you can expect labour to start on, or around, your due date. This will usually have been confirmed by an ultrasound scan in the early part of pregnancy, between 18 and 22 weeks. Being a biological event there is considerable variation however, and on a first birth in particular, it is not unusual for the pregnancy to go beyond the due date. In most cases if you are 10 or 12 days overdue you will either be monitored with ultrasound or offered induction of labour (see Chapter 7).

Has labour started?

The most characteristic feature of labour is painful contractions. If you are not getting regular, painful contractions at least every 8 minutes you can take it you are not in labour. Time your contractions from the beginning of one to the beginning of the next. If it is your first baby you may be confused between Braxton Hicks' ('practice') contractions and labour contractions. The strength of a labour pain is such that it will stop you in your tracks so that you have to grip on to something, you will not be able to talk through it, and if you are asleep, labour pains will wake you. They usually last at least 30 seconds. If you can walk, talk, eat, or sleep during a contraction it is unlikely to be a labour pain.

Not infrequently you will get episodes that make you think labour is starting, only for them to fade away after an hour or so. This tends to occur most often in the week or so before labour actually starts.

Strong supportive evidence that labour is starting is if the pains are accompanied by either a show, or the waters drain. A show is the coming away of the mucous plug that occupies the cervix and acts as a protective mechanism against infection from the birth canal. A typical show, when released, is blood stained. On its own a show does not mean labour has started, it only indicates this when it is accompanied by painful contractions.

Similarly if the waters drain, or 'go', in association with pains it is likely that labour is starting. The waters are usually clear, like tap water, and are usually released initially in a sudden gush and then continue to drain more slowly. A light greenish tinge, meconium staining, is unlikely to be sinister, especially if there is a good volume of fluid released.

If your waters drain but you have no contractions, you are not in labour, but you should make your way into the hospital without any great urgency. Delivery needs to take place within 72 hours of the waters draining in order to avoid infection. Once it has been confirmed that your waters are draining you may be advised to stay in hospital or you may prefer to rest at home and return next day to have your labour started (induction). If your waters have drained before 37 weeks you will probably be kept in hospital and receive antibiotics. When you reach 37 or 38 weeks your labour will probably be induced.

The initial contractions, show and natural rupture of the membranes usually take place over the course of 2–3 hours, though many different variations are possible in a healthy mother. However, most women who are going into labour for the first time will find they are only 1 cm dilated when they first go to hospital regardless of how long their contractions have lasted prior to leaving home.

Because the duration of labour tends to be longer in a first birth, you can expect to spend more time on the labour ward and may require more pain relief than on your next baby. Furthermore, your uterus may get tired and require assistance in delivering. The best measure of progress in labour is the rate of dilatation, or opening of the cervix. If your cervix is slow to dilate on a first labour, you may require oxytocin to be administered

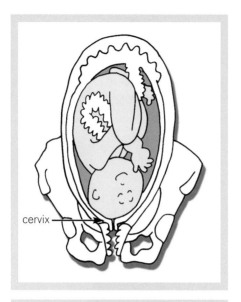

1 The cervix before labour is long, closed, and firm in texture.

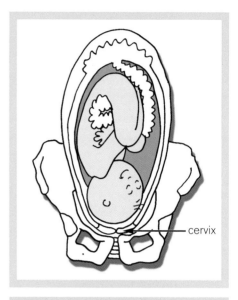

2 Effaced at the beginning of labour, the cervix has no length, admits a finger tip and is softer in texture.

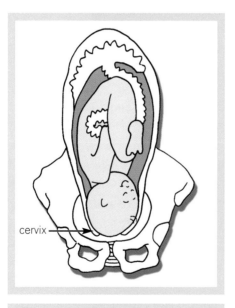

3 The cervix partly dilated

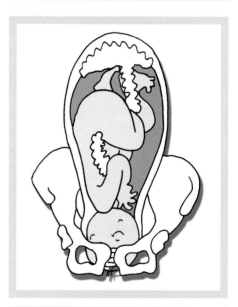

4 The cervix is fully dilated and there is a continuous passage from the top of the uterus to the outside world. Note the baby's head descending behind the pubic symphysis.

by drip to increase artificially the strength of your contractions and get you back on track. A graph plotting the course, and rate, of your dilatation will be updated after each vaginal examination during your labour.

Vaginal examination

When you arrive at hospital, the midwives will help settle you in and update your chart. You will not be shaved or given an enema and you can have a partner with you at all times if you choose. The midwives will perform an internal vaginal exam to see if you are in labour, and if so, how dilated you are. This procedure is the only way to assess your progress in labour and will usually be performed soon after you arrive in hospital and approximately every two hours thereafter during the first stage of labour. The purpose of the first vaginal examination is to diagnose whether or not your labour has started, by assessing the cervix, or neck of the womb. The examination is also useful to confirm that your baby is coming head first and to determine how far down in the pelvis your baby's head is.

Two things are examined. The first is the length of the cervix, the second the extent of its dilatation. As labour begins, the cervix shortens, or effaces, and then dilates. If your cervix has begun to dilate and you are getting regular, painful contractions at least every 8 minutes, labour has started.

On a first labour, the cervix begins to dilate after it has completely effaced (see figures opposite). In subsequent labours, effacement and dilatation can take place simultaneously, but diagnosis of labour is much easier because you as a mother are less likely to be mistaken about whether or not you are in labour.

Before labour starts, the cervix is closed and uneffaced; by the time you are ready to deliver there will be a continuous passage from the top of the uterus to the outside world. The measurements used to describe the amount of dilatation are approximate because every cervix is different, but a fully effaced cervix has a nominal measurement of 1 cm, a fully dilated cervix a nominal measurement of 10 cm.

show time

Often, the first sign that something is beginning to happen is a bloody show—a discharge of mucous mixed with blood. The show is often discharged when proper contractions first start but may appear 24 hours before labour begins in earnest. A small amount of blood or brown discharge may appear in advance of the show but this is not a sign that labour is beginning.

Particularly in a first labour, you may be disappointed to learn that your cervix has not opened any further or very little between examinations, despite your pains becoming much stronger. Don't be discouraged—a first labour is often slow to get going.

In a normal first labour you will have one exam to confirm that labour has begun. Immediately after that exam, your membranes may be ruptured (your waters will be broken) if they haven't gone already. There is no advantage to keeping the waters intact, indeed not having the waters broken could slow your labour significantly. Your second

The main difference between first and subsequent labours is duration. First labours are 50 per cent longer primarily because the uterus has not delivered a baby before and the cervix and birth canal have not been stretched. After you have delivered one baby, the uterus tends to work more efficiently and the cervix and birth canal stretch and dilate with much less resistance. The same holds true for the perineum and this explains why all forms of intervention, including stitches and episiotomies are much more common in first deliveries.

exam will probably be about two hours later and is to assess how much your cervix has dilated since admission. Your third exam is usually to confirm that your cervix has fully dilated if you have had oxytocin, or to assess your progress if you haven't had oxytocin.

You should expect to have not more than four or five exams in a normal first labour. If there are other problems, however, like the need for a blood sample to assess your baby's condition, there will obviously be more exams. On a second or subsequent labour you will probably need only two or three assessments as your labour is likely to be a lot quicker than your first.

The first stage of labour

On a first birth, the first stage of labour, (from when the cervix starts to dilate to when it is fully dilated) lasts an average of 6–7 hours. In subsequent births it may take only 3 or 4 hours or even less. At the end of the first stage the birth canal is a continuous passage from the top of the uterus to the outside world.

About 3 per cent of women will be in labour for more than 12 hours. The definition of prolonged labour varies from institution to institution but in Ireland a prolonged labour is one that sees the mother in the delivery ward for more than 12 hours. A substantial number of women deliver less than 6 hours after their admission to hospital. Within 4–5 hours of admission, you should have a reasonable idea of how long your labour will last, based on the rate of your dilatation. Midwives will be able to predict reasonably well how long a labour will last after their third examination.

If labour is not progressing on a first birth it is advisable to have contractions strengthened by the use of oxytocin. This undoubtedly will make contractions stronger and more intense but it is remarkably effective at speeding things up when used properly.

The duration of a second or subsequent labour is usually much shorter and on average lasts less than 4 hours from admission. Frequently, a second labour is over within an hour or two of arrival at the hospital. Many women are pleasantly surprised by the radical difference between their first and second births. Some women find the speed of developments almost overwhelming, particularly if the labour is too fast for an epidural to be effective, but are somewhat consoled by the fact that everything is over so much faster. It is unlikely that you will require oxytocin on a second or subsequent labour.

Pain relief

Labour is a painful process, but experiences differ enormously from woman to woman and labour to labour. The important thing to remember is that labour pain is a productive pain and persists only until the baby is born. The intense pain stops as soon as a contraction ends (so you will have some respite from it, even during a birth without pain relief) and disappears for good as soon as the baby is born. There is no doubt that the pain of labour is aggravated by fear of the unknown, so it is important to learn as much as possible about it, through antenatal classes, reading and discussion. When it comes to choosing pain relief, knowledge really is power.

During the first stage of labour you will need to make some decisions about pain relief. It is best to be flexible and open-minded about the various options available to you. It is all well and good to have a birth plan ready before you go into labour, but until you have actually felt what your contractions are like, you cannot know what is best for you and what you are capable of tolerating. You will not be doing yourself any favours if you are completely fixated on one kind of pain relief and cannot have it for medical reasons. If, for example, you are determined to have an epidural but arrive at the hospital nearly fully dilated, you must be prepared to find an acceptable alternative. Likewise, if you would like to have a drug-free childbirth but find that the pain is too much for you to cope with or your labour is prolonged, you should be open to accepting conventional pain relief.

There are many forms of pain relief available and what suits you and your labour is largely up to you. It is not at all unusual for a woman who has had three children to have opted for completely different types each time. This makes sense—her needs will differ every time and her past experiences will naturally influence her decisions. Also, different types of pain relief are fashionable at different times and new kinds are constantly being developed, so that what's popular varies tremendously from country to country as well as woman to woman. In Italy and Holland, for example, childbirth without epidural is the norm, whereas in Ireland more than 60 per cent of first-time mothers choose to have an epidural during their labour.

just so fast the second time

'My first labour lasted 13 hours but those hours flew so when my second baby was born in just under 2 hours I was kind of overwhelmed by how fast everything happened. My son was born at lunchtime but I was still totally pumped up at ten that night and had to take a sleeping pill to calm down. I didn't have time to get an epidural because I was already 7 cm dilated when I arrived in hospital and the anaesthetist was busy. I panicked at first even though I had wanted to try to give birth naturally. I guess being told there was no choice was scary. The midwives were obviously well used to this reaction because they knew just what to say and kept telling me I was doing great and the whole thing would be over in no time. They showed me how to use the gas and helped me with my breathing (but I have to say I think if you manage to breathe at all in any way you're winning)!'

the three stages of labour

1 From when the cervix begins to dilate to when it is fully dilated
2 From full dilatation to delivery of the baby
3 The delivery of the afterbirth, or placenta

Epidural

The most popular form of pain relief is the epidural anaesthetic. Epidurals are 99 per cent effective and provide excellent pain relief with virtually no risk, despite modern legends about paralysis. Many women find an epidural transforms the birthing experience completely—from a painful and frightening one to a pleasant, manageable one. Epidurals do not cause an increase in frequency of low back pain. This is due to the strain of pregnancy on your back, the physical exertion of delivery, and of course, lifting the baby afterwards.

The procedure itself involves the injection of a small amount of local anaesthetic into the small space surrounding the spinal cord. Doing so blocks the pain sensation in the lower half of the body but it may not fully block feelings of pressure or muscular movement (you may still be able to move your legs). In most cases, the mother feels almost completely numb from the waist down. Medication is given continuously through a pump mechanism in order to maintain steady pain relief.

walk on

Walking will not necessarily speed up labour but it may make you feel more comfortable in the early stages. Most hospitals don't mind if you walk around designated parts of the labour ward and many actively encourage it.

In theory, you may opt for an epidural as soon as it has been confirmed that you are in labour, although some hospitals and doctors may defer it until you are at least 4–5 cm dilated because it can slow the progress of labour. Others have no such reservations. Check with your doctor about the policy at your hospital.

If you are fully dilated or almost fully dilated, it is usually inadvisable to have an epidural. It would be too difficult for you to stay still while it was put into place. The good news in this situation is that if you are nearly fully dilated, the end to the pain is firmly in sight because delivery cannot be far off.

What to expect from an epidural

An anaesthetist will be summoned, which may take some time at night or if the hospital is busy. He or she will ask you to lie on your side or sit with your back towards them. Your back will be cleaned with antiseptic and a local anaesthetic will be given to numb the area so a fine needle can be passed through into the epidural space without you feeling it. It is essential that you lie absolutely still during this procedure because it is a delicate one and success depends on the anaesthetist knowing where the needle is by touch.

Once the needle is in place, a test dose of anaesthetic is infused to make sure you have no adverse reaction to it. Then, a very fine catheter will be fed through the needle into the epidural space so that medication can be infused through it for the remainder of labour.

The catheter will be taped into place and you should feel the lower part of your body go numb within minutes. You may be asked to turn from side to side to try and get an even spread of medication. Sometimes, women complain that one side of their body is more numb than the other, even after they turn. The epidural catheter will be removed after delivery and before you go to the post-natal ward. You will also require an IV drip with your epidural and this will restrict your movement further. This will also be removed before transfer to a post-natal ward.

If the epidural is in place longer than three hours, your bladder will need to be emptied to avoid over-stretching it because you will lose the sensation of needing to urinate. The nurse or midwife will place a catheter into the urethra every 2–3 hours during labour, and after the birth before you go to the post-natal ward, to ensure your bladder is empty.

Once the medication has ceased to be infused, the epidural wears off within an hour. You may need assistance when you first stand up, although you will normally be able to stand and get out of bed after 3–4 hours and regain full mobility within 12 hours.

Advantages
- Excellent, comprehensive relief from all painful sensations in the lower body
- Extremely low risk of complications
- No effect on baby

Disadvantages
- Mobility impaired during and after labour
- May make labour slightly longer
- May increase the need for forceps or vacuum delivery as pushing can be less effective in stage two of labour
- May increase the chances of delivery by caesarean section, depending on your hospital's policy on caesareans
- May induce a severe headache immediately after delivery when the mother sits up, due to leakage of spinal fluid. This happens in less than 1 per cent of cases and is remedied by injecting a small amount of the patient's own blood into the epidural space.
- Extra expense—an epidural costs several hundred euro extra if you are attending as a private patient.

next time, I'll do without drugs

'I wanted to have childbirth without drugs but after I had been in labour for about 8 hours and was really tired the midwife convinced me that I wasn't doing myself any favours by trying to cope with the pain so I had an epidural. It was a huge relief but I hated all the wires and tubes, especially the catheter for emptying my bladder. It felt like there were things taped to me everywhere. Next time, I'm determined to try and get through without it.'

running on empty

During labour the stomach does not empty, so eating during labour is discouraged. In fact, I've never come across a woman who wanted to eat during labour. If you have had a big meal just before labour starts, your meal will not be digested so you are more liable to vomit, particularly when the stomach drops following the birth of the baby. It is fine to drink water during labour, but drinking too much may also make you feel nauseated.

Spinal anaesthetic

The procedure and effect of the spinal anaesthetic is very like that of the epidural from the patient's point of view, but the anaesthetic is injected into the spine in a slightly different place. This type of anaesthetic is rarely used with a woman who has gone into labour. Medication is administered once rather than continuously, providing dense, almost complete pain relief. Many caesarean sections are performed using spinal anaesthesia.

Advantages
- Speed of pain relief is almost as fast as general anaesthesia, but it is safer

Disadvantages
- Sometimes causes low blood pressure and nausea

Walking epidural

Largely experimental, walking epidurals enable you to continue to walk during labour. Slightly less medication is given (just enough to dull the sensations of pain) but getting the dosage precisely right is difficult and balance is inevitably affected.

Pethidine

The most commonly used form of pain relief after the epidural, is the narcotic pethidine. It is given by intramuscular injection, usually in the buttock and ideally more than an hour before delivery. In long labours, it is not advisable to have too many injections as a large single or cumulative dose will often cause nausea and vomiting. In these circumstances, an anti-nausea drug will also be prescribed in tandem. Large doses may also cause the baby to be born sleepy or even partially sedated. It will take several days for the drug to be worked out of the baby's system.

In lower doses, pethidine often has the effect of making women feel detached from their pain although it does not remove the pain completely. If it does not cause nausea and vomiting, it is unlikely to cause the baby to be sedated.

Advantages
- Does not require an intravenous drip
- Allows you to walk around

Disadvantages
- May not remove pain completely
- Large doses may sedate the baby
- May make you sick

Gas and air through a face mask

A combination of oxygen and nitrous oxide self-administered through a face mask (or mouthpiece) in a way similar to that demonstrated in airline safety procedures is usually used as a short-term method of pain relief towards the end of the first stage of labour before pushing starts. The mask may make you feel quite confused and so make pushing effectively more difficult. The timing is also difficult to master under the conditions—you must inhale the gas as the contraction builds, then exhale and coast on the contraction as it dies down from its peak. Long, deep breaths rather than shallow sips or desperate gulps achieve the best results. Medication aside, it is useful as a distraction from the rigours of labour. Simply trying to concentrate on getting the most out of it focuses the mind and lets you take more control of the situation. Many women who have used both pethidine and the mask say they found the mask more effective.

Advantages
- No ill effect on baby
- Can stop taking it whenever you want
- The effects wear off fairly fast

Disadvantages
- May make you feel confused
- Can be difficult to self-administer
- Only takes the edge off the pain

The TENS machine

The TENS machine, which is available in chemists, stimulates the nerves under the skin with vibrating pulses. It looks more or less like a Walkman with a few wires connected to sticky patches. The patches are stuck on to your back and then you control the intensity of the pulses yourself by turning a dial. Most people start using it too late on in labour and so compromise its effectiveness. It must be used as soon as labour begins, exactly as described in the instruction book. Many women find it gives some relief but is increasingly less effective as labour progresses.

Advantages
- No ill effect on baby
- Non-invasive and drug-free
- Self-administered

Disadvantages
- Must begin at the onset of labour to be very effective
- Recent studies have questioned its effectiveness
- Cost of rental

TENS

'I used the TENS machine when my labour started more or less to help avoid going to hospital as long as possible. At first I was using a pretty low setting and getting by fine—if I pushed up the intensity it felt really unpleasant. After a couple of hours the dial was all the way at the top and I couldn't feel the pulses at all. That was when I knew it was definitely time to go to hospital. When I got there I was 7 cm dilated and well on my way. So as far as I'm concerned it worked.'

You will probably choose someone to come with you to provide emotional support during labour. Most people choose to have their partner present and depend on the hospital to provide additional professional support. Others find that a close friend or relative who has given birth herself can give the best emotional support and practical advice. If your partner does not feel comfortable being at the birth you should try to understand his feelings and remember that his discomfort may also make you uncomfortable when the chips are down. The last thing you need when you are working through a strong contraction is to be worried about how your partner is bearing up. Likewise, when you are concentrating on pushing you don't need someone flitting around trying to mop your brow and looking seriously worried. It could be that you would be better off with your mother or sister at your side or relying only on professional support. Whereas in the last few decades, most fathers used to attend the birth as a matter of course, there is now a growing contingent who choose to wait outside the delivery ward during labour. It's completely up to you and your partner to decide how you handle this aspect of your labour.

Relaxation techniques

At antenatal classes you will learn breathing and relaxation techniques to help you relax and cope with the pain of labour. If you keep focused on the baby's imminent arrival and concentrate on finding the inner reserves to deal with the pain you may find that you can cope with the enormity of labour without having any drugs. A birthing partner or coach can train with you at antenatal classes to learn the most effective ways of controlling breathing and staying calm throughout labour. Even if you are planning to have an epidural, learning relaxation techniques for the earliest stages of labour can be a great help to you, both in managing your pain and in making the experience more positive.

A single trained professional, a midwife or student midwife will probably accompany you throughout labour. She will help guide you through various relaxation and breathing techniques. This is a great advantage as it allows your husband or partner to relax and not feel any weight of responsibility for how you are feeling and coping with the stress of labour.

In the first stage of labour you will be encouraged to take long, deep breaths and to exhale them slowly during contractions. In the second stage you will be pushing in time with your contractions. Your midwife will talk you through practically every breath and will be a tremendous support to you.

Hypnosis

Hypnosis is very rarely used in labour and is probably not a very good idea as you will not be in touch with what is happening and what you are feeling.

Water

Many women find taking a shower or bath is a good way to help relieve pain during labour. However, it is not possible to monitor the condition of your baby properly in either. I would advise strongly against giving birth in a bath, or 'birthing pool'. There is no evidence that humans have ever given birth in this way. It is completely unnatural, to say nothing of the risk to your baby. Many babies take a breath, and some even cry, once the head is outside the birth canal and there are well-documented cases of babies drowning as a consequence of being delivered in a birthing pool.

The second stage of labour

The second stage of labour begins when the cervix is fully dilated and ends with the birth of the baby. In a first birth it usually lasts from 40 to 60 minutes. In a second, and subsequent birth it is much shorter and is sometimes over in a matter of 10 minutes or less.

This part of labour is usually taken up completely with pushing, which can be difficult to get right on a first baby. If you have not had an epidural, you will usually feel an overwhelming physical desire to push as soon as you are fully dilated and your body will more or less tell you what to do. You will be in no doubt about whether it's time to push or not. If you have had an epidural, the midwife will tell you when to begin pushing as you may not feel the strong urge to bear down. You should push as if you are severely constipated—the direction of push is the same. Each push helps the uterine contraction move the baby further down the birth canal. It is important to time your pushing in concert with contractions. Your midwife or doctor will help coach you—listen to their advice about when to push so as not to tire yourself out with unproductive effort.

If you have had an epidural, following this advice is even more important because the epidural may suppress your urge to push, making timing more problematic. It is always best to wait until the midwife and doctor tell you to push because sometimes you may feel like pushing before the baby's head has descended completely or before you are fully dilated. If you push before you should, you may injure your cervix. Sometimes the density of epidural may be allowed to diminish so that you have some sensation of pressure in your pelvis to help you know when to push.

On a first baby, the pushing phase is generally over within an hour. If you are pushing for an hour and delivery is still not imminent, it is likely that you will need assistance with delivery either by forceps or vacuum. In a small number of cases, if the head does not descend sufficiently, a caesarean section is necessary. You will probably have approximately 12 to 15 contractions in an hour so the average first baby will require 36–45 pushes to be delivered. This is hard physical work ('labour'!) so that you will probably be tired and stiff for a few days afterwards, as if you had gone running for an hour when you were unfit.

On second or subsequent labours, pushing is usually over within 20–30 minutes. You will probably manage three pushes with each contraction, with contractions in the second stage usually no more than 5 minutes apart. On a second or subsequent birth a lot fewer pushes will be required—sometimes no more than two or three during one contraction.

If it looks like your perineum will not stretch enough or if there is any suspicion of foetal distress and labour needs to be shortened at this stage, an episiotomy will be done just before the baby's head is delivered when the perineum is really stretched. A perineum

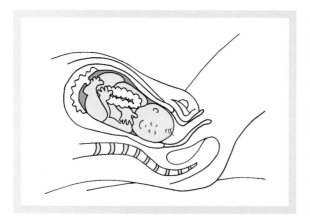

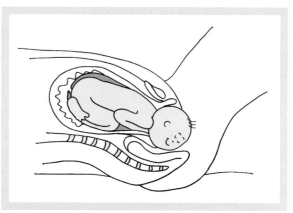

1 The cervix is now fully dilated and there is a continuous passage from the uterus to the outside world.

2 The top of the baby's head has now emerged and can be seen.

that does not stretch may delay delivery by 20 minutes or more. There is no evidence that perineal massage lessens the likelihood that you will either tear or require an episiotomy.

Birth positions

Usually, the mother is propped up in a semi-sitting position for the actual birth. Almost no one lies flat on their back or opts for a more unusual position. Squatting or kneeling on all fours confers no advantage, gravitational or otherwise. In fact, these positions make it much more difficult for medical staff to see what's going on and to help accordingly. Birthing chairs, which enjoyed a brief vogue in the 1980s, are associated with more stitches and a higher incidence of post partum haemorrhage and so have been largely abandoned.

Lying on the side is also a common and effective position. Whatever feels most comfortable to you is best.

Delivery

As delivery of the baby's head takes place, you will be asked to stop pushing and pant. This helps minimise tearing of the perineum or extending an episiotomy by exerting too much pressure too quickly on it. After delivery of the baby's head there will usually be a gap of a few minutes until the next contraction. During this hiatus, the baby's nose and mouth may be sucked out as a precaution. If there is meconium present, this helps stop the baby swallowing it, amniotic fluid, mucous and blood.

With the next contraction, you will be asked to give another strong push to deliver the baby's shoulders and body. Once the shoulders are clear, the body slithers out easily.

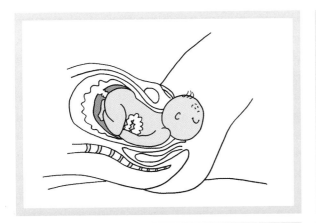

3 The baby's head has emerged further.

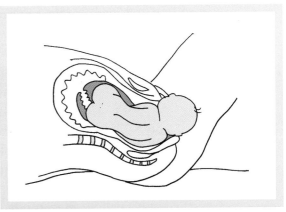

4 Now the baby has turned, and the head is fully born.

A feeling of profound physical relief usually coincides with your first sight of the baby.

The baby will probably be a deep purple colour initially, particularly above the neck. This is normal. It is due to a process known as auto regulation of blood flow, whereby the most important organs in the body are supplied with oxygen first. The baby's first breath is usually taken almost immediately, definitely within the first minute of birth and the purple will turn to pink in a few minutes as breathing becomes established. Your baby will be covered in a mixture of blood, liquor, vernix and possibly meconium, and may blow bubbles when he or she

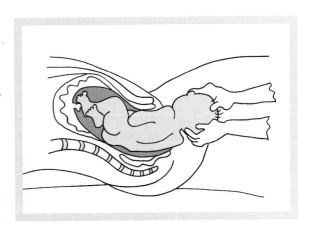

5 The baby is gently assisted out into the world.

breathes while clearing fluid from the lungs. Not all babies cry loudly or at all at birth, some are mellow and just breathe quietly. Both are perfectly normal. Your baby may blink in the bright light, having just emerged from darkness. Most babies stretch (not surprising considering they're coming from a very tight space) and may kick vigorously. At birth the baby's head may be elongated because it has moulded to the shape of the birth canal—it will quickly return to normal.

The baby is usually placed on your tummy to your breast and covered with a warm towel, as heat is lost quickly your baby will feel as you do after emerging from a hot shower into a cool room. Your tummy is then checked for an undiagnosed twin (most unusual these days!) and an injection is given into your thigh to help speed delivery of the placenta. Name bracelets will be placed on the baby, and the umbilical cord will be clamped and cut. After you have had a few minutes together, your baby will be taken for weighing and a quick examination by the midwife and will be given an Apgar score.

The Apgar score, named after Virginia Apgar, an American anaesthetist, was developed in 1952. It is a method of assessing the condition of the baby in the minutes after birth using heart rate, breathing, colour, muscle tone and movement, and response to stimulation. The score is usually taken at one and five minutes after delivery. The usual score is 9 at one minute and 10 at five minutes. Babies are usually more purple than pink at delivery because the blood circulating just beneath the skin has to pass through the newly opened lungs to become pink and then circulate back to the skin again, hence the delay and deduction of one point in the Apgar score for a normal baby. The Apgar score does not indicate whether or not a baby is low in oxygen at birth and does not correlate well with future development. So, if your baby has a low Apgar score at either one or five minutes this does not inevitably mean that the baby was deprived of oxygen.

A complete examination by a paediatrician takes place within a day or two. In some hospitals a security tag similar to a shoplifting tag will be attached to your baby's ankle. This is to safeguard against your baby being taken from the hospital.

The third stage of labour

The third stage of labour refers to delivery of the placenta or afterbirth. After you have delivered your baby, assisted by the midwives, there is an interval before the placenta delivers—usually within 10 to 15 minutes. An injection of syntometrine helps the uterus to contract and assists with making delivery of the placenta easier. The injection also helps to reduce the amount of bleeding from your uterus. Some women prefer to let the baby's cord stop pulsing and to attempt to breastfeed in an effort to make the third stage as physiologically normal as possible. There are no great advantages to be had however, and it is probably simpler not to delay.

While the baby is being examined, the placenta will usually have separated and become ready for delivery. The doctor or midwife will press on your stomach and pull on the umbilical cord until the placenta is expelled. The cord, or lifeline, of the baby is redundant after the baby is born and has begun to breathe. It may still pulse briefly after the baby is born but after a few minutes the baby's circulation is established and placental circulation stops. You may be interested to see and touch the cord—it is a remarkable piece of engineering, consisting of two blood vessels to the placenta and one coming back. These vessels are heavily insulated by a thick rubbery substance called Wharton's jelly, which prevents the blood vessels from compressing even if they are wrapped around the baby's neck. If you or your partner cut the cord, it will be shockingly tough, like gristle.

The placenta looks like a large liver, and although not much to look at, it is an amazing organ that has sustained your baby for its entire life in utero. The midwife or doctor will check that it has been delivered in its entirety, because any missing bits retained in the womb could precipitate infection or bleeding. If the placenta has not been fully delivered it may need to be removed under anaesthetic.

If you need stitches they will be done now under local anaesthetic. If you have had an epidural, it will provide complete relief and you won't need a local. The stitches usually take only a few minutes and surprisingly, are not very uncomfortable going in. Many a woman who has dreaded stitches more than any part of labour barely notices she's having them. IV drips and the epidural will be removed within the hour and the midwife will help you tidy up before transfer to the post-natal ward. You and your partner will also be offered light refreshments and a phone to call friends and relatives.

You should put your baby to the breast within an hour of birth—the midwife in the labour ward will help you. Babies often get a bit sleepy later, they're tired too.

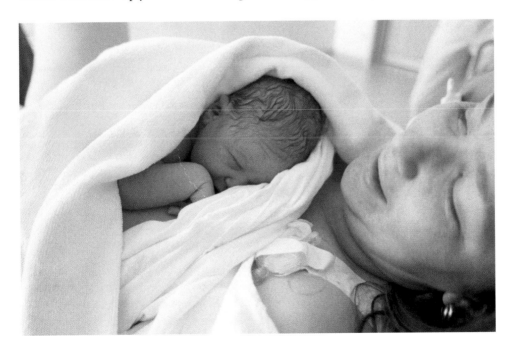

unplanned home birth

If your labour starts at home and progresses much faster than you expected you may be faced with the prospect of giving birth at home. This is extremely unlikely on a first birth, indeed I cannot remember such a birth in all my time in practice. So, if this is your first pregnancy don't worry—it is most unlikely to happen! If it does happen, here's what to do:

1 Don't panic.

2 Phone the ambulance service and tell them what's happening. They've seen it before and they are well trained to deal with the situation. Phone number: 999 or 112.

3 Gather some towels and go to the kitchen.

4 Spread out the towels and lie on them, but keep one large one to wrap the baby in.

5 When you feel the baby's head coming place your hand over it to try and slow its exit; try to control the speed of delivery so that the baby's head eases out rather than 'shoots' out. Don't worry if you don't succeed in this as your baby won't be harmed but you may tear yourself.

6 When your baby's head has emerged take a breather and wait for the next contraction. During this time your baby will turn its head to one side. This can be pretty uncomfortable but is normal.

7 Just before the final contraction your baby may give a little kick or squirmy movement. There may also be a rush of fluid with the beginning of the last contraction.

8 You may need to push hard to complete the delivery; if there seems to be a delay, pull your thighs up against your abdomen/chest and push again.

9 If there is someone to help they should grip the baby's head at the start of the last contraction and pull down gently towards your rectum as you push.

10 The baby will probably emerge in a rush of fluid and blood, give a startled look, make a face, throw open his or her arms and roar. Remember, babies usually look purple when they emerge so don't be frightened by the appearance. As long as your baby is breathing you need have no concerns, they don't always cry.

11 Wrap your baby up well with the big towel you have kept for this purpose. The biggest problem babies born unexpectedly at home have is getting too cold—hypothermia.

12 The umbilical cord. You can either tie it off with two bits of string, or shoe laces, and cut between the two knots, or you can wait. It will stop pulsating itself and no harm is done to the baby, or mother, by waiting.

13 Have a cup of tea, you deserve it!

Unexpected home birth is very uncommon in my experience. Much more frequent is where a woman comes to hospital and gives birth within minutes of arrival. There are also those who deliver in the ambulance on the way. So, despite apocryphal stories that your 'friends' may tell you about the speed of second births, it is very unlikely to happen to you.

in the bag

When you first head into hospital, don't take everything you'll need for the entire stay. Bring just what you'll need for the first night and day after and leave valuables at home. One overnight bag should get you and your baby through the first night. Visitors can bring in clean clothes (and take away dirty clothes) and save you the hassle of making sure they get from the delivery ward to the post-natal ward (and possibly more than one room change).

You should have in your bag:

T-shirt or short nightdress to wear during labour

Slippers or slip-on shoes for walking in the halls during labour

Dressing gown

A good sized towel for bathing after delivery

12 sanitary towels—heavy flow

Toiletries (shampoo, soap, toothbrush, toothpaste, make-up)

Nightdress or pyjamas, to change into after delivery

Old knickers/disposable panties

Laundry bag

Camera

Hairdryer

Glasses (if you wear contact lenses you may need to take them out)

Nursing bra

Any medications you may need for asthma, etc.

5–6 baby vests and babygros, and a towel for the baby

20 newborn size nappies

Wipes or cotton wool and lotion

Sudocrem/Vaseline

A book or magazine

And perhaps . . .

This book

Tissues

Snacks for your partner if it's the middle of the night

Mobile phone

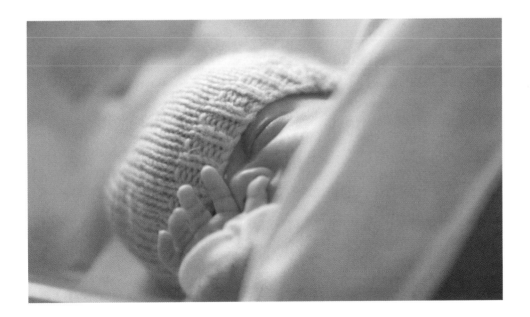

a birth at the National Maternity Hospital Dublin
from Mothering the Mother, by Klaus, Kennell and Klaus, Perseus Books 1993

The authors spent a week observing women in labour at the National Maternity Hospital and found that the midwives there were a 'model of humane care'.

The following scene was typical of many we observed. The mother and father arrive at the hospital. The mother has been having contractions, and she thinks she is in labour. The midwife in charge greets her, helps her get comfortable, puts her in the examining room and invites the father to come in or wait in the waiting room. As the mother has a contraction, the midwife gently but clearly starts her guiding instructions, even before examining the mother. 'Lie on your side, breathe in through your nose, and long slow breaths out through your mouth. Keep your eyes open; look at me—good, keep doing that, nice and slowly, that's good (she models for her). Purse your lips, make a swish sound as you breathe out—good. Take a big breath in through your nose, keep your eyes open—look at the window or at my face, blow and release, breathe out through your mouth. Again; now look at me, that keeps your mind off the pain. That's right, you're doing great, you're doing marvellous. What time did the pain start? ' The mother says she had pains all night. 'Did you sleep?' She dozed. 'Was there a bloody show?' Yesterday, she indicates. 'How much blood? Show me in my hand.' The midwife explains everything before she does it. 'I'm going to examine you to see if you're in labour. If you are, I'm going to break the bag of waters to check the colour of the water and to accelerate the labour. Okay? Tell me when you are getting a pain. Now I'll set you up and tell you what's happening.' (She has checked the mother's pulse, blood pressure and temperature.) She examines the mother. 'You're in labour—three centimetres, a very good start. I haven't broken the waters yet because the baby's head is not yet down. I want you to walk for one hour. Walking helps get the head down. Walk with your husband and the nurse now. The best way to get the baby's head down is by walking. Then it'll be very quick. I think you'll have a short labour. I'll examine you later.' She introduces the mother to her personal nurse-midwife.

The three of them proceed slowly down the corridor. The nurse-midwife almost always has her hand on the mother. It is quiet, peaceful and calm. They pass a similar trio. The nurse-midwife says, 'Tell me when you feel a contraction starting—we'll stop and I'll help you through it.' The woman says, 'Yes, now.' They stop; the nurse-midwife suggests that the woman lean easily against the wall, and she helps her through the contraction. The time passes quickly in this fashion: they walk, they listen and as contractions get stronger or the mother feels any change or wants to get in bed, the nurse-midwife follows at the mother's pace; staying with her for every moment of the experience, reassuring, validating, comforting, appropriately respecting the father's position, and being the stable presence of experience and confidence for both the mother and the father.

The midwife in charge comes periodically throughout the labour to help the training nurse-midwife who is providing support. She checks what is happening, reassures the mother, and at appropriate times checks for dilatation. As the second stage gets under way (when the cervix is fully dilated and the head is descending), many women sometimes lose their sense of direction and control. They feel overwhelmed and even having delivered several children may say, 'I can't do it. No, it's really too hard—I can't do it!' At this point both midwives help the woman in pushing the baby out, with the charge midwife reminding the mother how to push through the contraction, but only when she feels like pushing. Here is an excellent example of how this intense one-to-one communication is essential. The nurse-midwife says softly, 'Just one person talking so as not to cause distraction. We're going to make use of that contraction. When it comes, let's use your own power to push this baby out. Good, good, take a deep breath—no talk or sound. Put your chin on your chest and push that breath into your bottom as long as you can hold it, then quickly two more times within this contraction. In three contractions you're going to push that baby right out. I can see its hair—great, good, you're doing great.'

'Now, rest in between contractions.' She helps the woman into position. Sometimes the mother gets leverage by holding her own knees, or the two midwives let the mother push her feet against them to brace herself. It was unusual for us to see such close physical contact—so much more humane than the old stirrups. The woman either sits up in the bed, as high as possible, or is on her left side. The midwives often use a bed-wedge pillow behind her back.

As the contraction starts, the nurse-midwife reminds the mother, 'We're going to make the best use of this pushing energy. Now another contraction: take a big breath, mouth closed, chin on chest, and push into your bottom and forward. Hold the breath as long as possible. Good, now a second big breath. Good, go along with the urge to push. Now a third big breath—good, push into your bottom and stay forward. Good, good, the baby's come forward a lot. You're great. Now rest. Let me know when the urge to push starts—that first push is the best push. Good.' She has the father stand just behind the mother with his arm around her shoulders, letting him support the mother as she pushes. The midwives recognise the mother's incredible need for encouragement in order to keep going. Even when any of the team or family is tired, the midwives keep going cheerfully, reminding the mother that she has all the power she needs to push the baby out and that she's feeling pressure now, not pain. When the head has crowned, the midwives guide the mother gently to relax and look at the focal point, just breathing in a light and slow breath to let her body do the rest of the natural pushing out of the baby . . .

Sitting as quiet observers in the corner of the room for an extended period, we saw an entire system geared toward supporting the mother and father through their baby's birth—without anxiety and with gentle caring, encouragement, warmth and displays of real affection.

After your baby is born

If delivery has occurred in the evening it will probably be very difficult to get any sleep without a sleeping tablet. You will be on a high, replaying events over and over in your mind at a fierce pace. Taking a mild sleeping tablet will not harm your baby if you are breastfeeding, and likewise, if you are prescribed painkillers for afterpains (particularly on a second or subsequent birth—see below), these will not affect the baby adversely.

Within the next 12 hours, you should recover your strength sufficiently to have a shower or bath on your own and receive visitors.

In the immediate post-natal period, you may feel overwhelmed by everything that has happened, particularly if you have just had your first baby. You may also be sore, a bit bruised and stiff or exhausted from having been on a high following the birth that kept you awake but within days of delivery you should be managing feeding, washing and the general care of your baby.

Stitches

If you have stitches, there is usually some swelling for a day or two after the birth that may make them pull slightly. If possible you should soak often in a bath with nothing added (no salts, antiseptics or oils). They should be much less sore within 3–4 days of delivery.

Breastfeeding

If you are breastfeeding, you will find your milk comes in during the first two to three days after delivery. Until you settle into feeding, your breasts may fill up dramatically and leak. There is usually some tenderness while feeding until you get used to it and have mastered proper positioning of the baby. The midwives will help you establish the correct position the first time you bring the baby to the breast and will attend you at subsequent feedings. Even if you have fed before, you may have forgotten how best to manage a newborn. Some babies do not take to feeding immediately after birth, others attack the breast with great gusto. The first time the baby clamps on will feel strange and surprisingly strong—the baby will take the whole areola into its mouth and suck with impressive force, often for as long as it is allowed. Since you will be unaccustomed to feeding, this first flirtation with it should not last too long or your nipples will quickly become sore. The baby may get a tiny bit of colostrum, or immunity-imparting pre-milk, at this first trip to the breast, but your milk will not begin to come in for at least 24 hours. Ask the midwife or doctor any questions as they arise. Breastfeeding does not just happen, however natural it is.

It takes two to three days to get breastfeeding established; it takes two weeks to get it going well, so be patient. The secret is—sleep when your baby sleeps and don't worry

are very important for you
This is a very special time
, you will be very tired for
al and you need plenty of
l if he/she could help with
and feed the baby.

ll not be sucking and stimulating your milk
for a day or two but they will then return to
mfort and tenderness. Wear a good supportive
op breast milk production.

he first three days after delivery and slowly
light. After you go home you may experience
xert yourself or breastfeed. As long as bleeding
every hour) you need not be concerned. You
od that has collected inside the uterus before
ignificance and there is no need to keep them
ay find that you also pass them when you have
h may also bring about a rush of bright red

n the third day after delivery. You may be very
aven't slept enough. These feelings generally
don't, you may be developing depression and
lling. Contact your GP initially and you will
ou prefer, you may also directly contact the
mportant thing about post-natal depression is
l can cause terrible problems for you and your
. While the causes of post-natal depression are
all.

> **contraception**
> Contrary to folklore, breast-feeding does not act as a contraceptive.

Afterpains

These are cramplike pains caused by the uterus contracting back to normal size after the birth. The pains are usually quite mild, like period cramps, after a first baby, but are often much more severe after subsequent births. They last only for the first few days following the birth. Prescribed pain killers will help you cope.

Frequently asked questions

Does the doctor have a good idea of what sex and size the baby will be?
Sex is impossible to guess despite folklore about the way a mother is carrying, but the doctor usually has a reasonably good idea of the approximate size of the baby. It is much more difficult to estimate a baby's size if you are overweight. Ultrasound estimation of fetal weight has a margin of error of at least 10 per cent.

How do you time contractions?
From the beginning of one until the beginning of the next.

I think I'm having contractions but all my pain seems concentrated in my back. I thought it would be over my tummy. Is this normal?
It is unusual but not abnormal. If your whole tummy is going hard the pains are contractions.

Is it better to have an episiotomy or a natural tear?
An episiotomy will usually only be performed if faster delivery is required or if a large tear is going to occur. A small tear is preferable to an episiotomy because it heals better, even if stitches are required.

If I have really strong tummy muscles will I be able to push more effectively?
Yes. Women who are fit usually have short labours.

Are there any exercises I can do to strengthen up the right muscles?
Not really after you get pregnant. Better to get fit beforehand and maintain your fitness throughout.

A friend has suggested I bring a doula with me to the hospital when I go into labour. What is a doula and is this a good suggestion?
A doula is a lay woman (not a nurse or midwife) who provides valuable psychological support in countries where there are not enough midwives. This does not apply in Ireland. The concept of the doula was introduced into Western obstetric practice by Doctors Klaus, Kennell and Klaus (see page 80). In Ireland midwives provide the same service as doulas so in this country it is not necessary to hire an extra person yourself.

7 interventions in labour

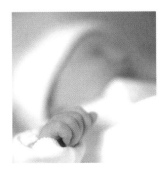

There are a variety of interventions in labour that you should be aware of, ranging from the simplest, like vaginal examination to assess your progress in labour, to the more complicated, like taking a sample of blood from your baby's scalp to assess his or her condition and ability to tolerate labour. The most extreme intervention is delivery by caesarean section, which is covered in Chapter 8. Many interventions are designed to assist you achieve a normal birth in a reasonable period of time, so that you are fit enough to care for your baby and do not feel completely exhausted by the whole birth process.

Common interventions

Common interventions in a first labour include vaginal examination, breaking the waters, the administration of intravenous fluids, epidural pain relief, intermittent drainage of your bladder by catheterisation, oxytocin infusion, episiotomy, stitches and less frequently, vacuum or forceps delivery. In subsequent labours, usual interventions are confined to vaginal examination and less frequently, epidural pain relief, which necessitates intravenous fluids. If you have a normal delivery on your first labour, subsequent labours are generally trouble-free.

Intervention on first vs. second births	First birth	Second birth
Vacuum	20%	2%
Caesarean section	15–30%	5–15%
Stitches	50%	20%

Breaking the waters

If your waters have not already leaked by themselves, which they do in about one-third of women, it is advisable to have them artificially broken. This procedure has the dual advantage of enabling your caregiver to see the colour and volume of the fluid around your baby, and helping your labour to progress. A normal flow of clear fluid is very reassuring with regard to your baby's health and, unless there is some unanticipated difficulty, means it is unlikely your baby will develop a problem in labour. There is no advantage to keeping your membranes intact, although on a second or subsequent birth your labour may progress rapidly with intact membranes. If you have already started labour naturally, artificially rupturing the membranes is not an induction of labour. However, if you have not yet gone into labour breaking the waters may induce it to start.

The procedure is done during a vaginal examination. The midwife passes a plastic device with a sharp hook at the end along her fingers and through the cervical opening. The membranes, like cling film, are ruptured by moving the hook back and forth. There is usually a gush of fluid to confirm the waters have been 'broken'.

Oxytocin

Oxytocin is a substance that is made naturally in your body. It acts specifically on your uterus in labour to cause contractions. Artificially produced oxytocin is commonly used in obstretics both to induce labour and to accelerate a labour that is progressing slowly. However, its use is a potent source of confusion. It is not a particularly successful drug for inducing labour (but then nothing is) but when used to accelerate a labour that has already begun, it is one of the most effective drugs available in modern medicine. Oxytocin is frequently used in a first birth to help progress and achieve a normal vaginal delivery but is seldom required on a second or subsequent birth. The reduced need for oxytocin on later births is due to the more efficient nature of a uterus that has already delivered and the fact that the lower genital tract has been stretched by previous deliveries.

If oxytocin is required to help your labour progress, it will be given intravenously through a drip. If you do not have an epidural there is no reason why you should not continue to walk around once it is administered. Dosage at first is low and is gradually increased in a step by step fashion, usually every 15 minutes. Your contractions will be stronger, possibly more frequent, and probably more painful.

Episiotomy

One of the fears of pregnant women is the thought of an episiotomy—the cut made in the perineum (the area between the vaginal opening and anus) if it becomes necessary to either hasten delivery or prevent a bad tear occurring during delivery (which may need stitches anyway). In the heat of labour, its importance usually pales considerably. If you have to have one (and most women don't) it is a relatively minor procedure and should only cause you some discomfort in the days following the birth, and none thereafter. It should heal quickly and thoroughly.

No one wants to have unnecessary stitches and discomfort, so you may want to check if your hospital's episiotomy rate is abnormally high. Make sure you ask for the rate in vaginal deliveries (excluding caesareans) as episiotomies are not performed with caesareans and the inclusion of caesareans in calculations will make the rate seem lower than it actually is.

avoiding an episiotomy

Some people feel that the best way to avoid an episiotomy is to massage the perineum with vitamin E cream or almond oil in the last month of pregnancy. However, research does not support this.

Episiotomies are no longer performed routinely in most hospitals, although they are almost inevitable if you have an instrumental delivery with vacuum or forceps. The procedure is much more common on a first birth. If you are having your first baby, you will have an approximately 50 per cent chance of requiring stitches either from an episiotomy or perineal tear; as the rate of episiotomy goes down, the rate of tear goes up! Look on the bright side, though—you have a 50 per cent chance of not having stitches, too. There is good evidence that a natural tear heals better than an episiotomy. For this reason, most doctors and midwives will avoid an episiotomy unless the perineum is too resistant and there is a danger of a large tear occurring or the perineum is unduly delaying the delivery process.

Before the episiotomy, you will be given a local anaesthetic if you don't have a well-functioning epidural already in place, so you will not feel it being done.

Foetal monitoring

Your baby and placenta are well adapted to tolerate the inherent stresses of labour; the human race would have died out long ago if this were not the case. If your baby is healthy when labour begins and if labour does not last too long, there is no reason to expect that the experience will have any ill effect on him or her. Ways of effectively monitoring your baby are really quite limited; they include listening to your baby's heart with a special stethoscope or electronically, and using a clip attached to the baby's scalp to monitor the pulse rate. However, there are certain observations that are generally helpful.

- A good size baby at term where labour starts spontaneously is off to a good start.
- The presence of a normal volume of amniotic fluid, particularly if it is clear, suggests that the placenta has been working well during the latter part of pregnancy.

During labour, your baby's heart rate and certain other characteristics will be monitored either continuously or intermittently. In some hospitals, all babies' heart rates are monitored continuously; others adopt a more selective approach. A normal heart rate means your baby is not suffering from a lack of oxygen. An abnormal heart rate does not necessarily mean your baby is suffering from a lack of oxygen, but the more abnormal the heart rate, the more likely there is to be a diminishing oxygen supply. Even with the most abnormal patterns, however, only a small proportion represent true 'foetal distress'.

The problem for the doctor is to determine which patterns represent oxygen deficiency. In order to clarify the situation, a sample of blood may be taken from the baby's scalp during a special vaginal examination. This foetal blood sample (FBS) determines whether or not your baby should be delivered by caesarean section or labour can safely be allowed to continue. The baby's heart rate pattern alone is usually too non-specific to dictate such an important decision. The FBS procedure may need to be repeated to determine a pattern or if delivery is not imminent. The decision about further management will depend on a number of circumstances including the colour and volume of amniotic fluid, the rate of progress in labour, the gestational age of the baby and whether the baby is felt to be suitably mature. The procedure of FBS is not practised in all hospitals.

Continuous electronic monitoring

This can be done externally by attaching a sensor disk to your abdomen with a big belt. The disk traces your baby's heartbeat. Internal monitoring is done by attaching a special clip to your baby's scalp during a vaginal examination. It feeds information about your baby's pulse rate into an electronic monitor.

Extensive research has been conducted to determine the benefits or otherwise of routine continuous electronic monitoring in low risk births. The research has shown that babies who are monitored continuously have a slightly decreased chance of suffering a seizure as newborns, a rare event in itself. In the long term, however, monitoring makes no difference to the chances of developing cerebral palsy and/or intellectual disability. Furthermore, routine monitoring has not been shown to reduce the chance of death in labour—a very rare event. Monitoring does however increase the chances that your delivery will be operative, either vacuum or forceps, or by caesarean section. This is because doctors will always err on the side of caution and deliver a baby who is showing heart rate changes that might indicate a reduced oxygen supply. Unfortunately, a perfectly healthy baby's heart rate behaves in a fairly bizarre way in many labours and this results in many unnecessary operative deliveries in the mistaken belief that a baby is distressed. It is of course safer to assume the baby may need help and an operative delivery where there is any doubt about the baby's health.

Assisted delivery with vacuum or forceps

There are really only two reasons for an assisted vaginal delivery with vacuum (ventouse) or forceps. The first is suspected foetal distress and the second is slow progress of the baby with pushing. Assisted vaginal delivery can only be performed in the second stage of labour; in the first stage, caesarean section is the only way to deliver a baby. If you are becoming exhausted and are unable to push your baby out yourself, you may need help. Forceps may also be used in breech delivery to assist in delivery of the baby's head in a controlled fashion.

The choice of whether to use vacuum or forceps is an individual one, and your doctor will decide which is most appropriate in the circumstances. There is some evidence that the vacuum may be less likely to damage the perineum than forceps but much research remains to be done to clarify this.

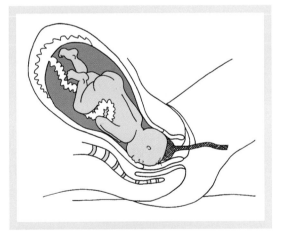

VACUUM ASSISTED DELIVERY

Vacuum or suction is used to assist delivery if it seems that the baby is distressed, or if there is slow progress with the delivery. In a vacuum assisted delivery a plastic or metal cup is attached to the baby's head and a vacuum is created by suction. The doctor pulls on the attached rubber tube in time with your contractions until the baby's head is delivered.

If you have an epidural you will need to have your bladder emptied artificially by the passage of a catheter. The reason for this is that the epidural suppresses the sensation of fullness that normally tells you to empty your bladder. If your bladder over-fills it can cause serious problems in future. Your bladder may be emptied either intermittently by your midwife, or continuously by an 'indwelling' catheter during labour.

On your first baby, your chances of needing assistance will range from 15 per cent to 30 per cent, depending on where you have your baby. Ask your doctor or midwife for the figures for their hospital. The incidence of assisted delivery is influenced by attitudes within the hospital and approaches to care in labour, and the differences in these can be pronounced.

On a second or subsequent birth, your chances of requiring assistance are greatly reduced. You may still have difficulty pushing, however, because of an epidural, because your baby is large, or because the contractions are not strong enough. Weak contractions can sometimes be corrected with oxytocin, which may be started for the first time in the second stage of labour if the baby's head is not descending with contractions. This judgment call will be made by a senior midwife or doctor.

Sometimes, an epidural will be allowed to wane in intensity during the second stage of labour so that you have some sensation of pressure in the pelvis with contractions to help you know when to push. This may help avoid the requirement for assistance. If it is suspected that your baby is showing signs of distress, a vacuum or forceps delivery is advisable to shorten the second stage of labour.

If you have been in labour for a long time, your baby's head may appear quite misshapen and perhaps 'cone-headed'. This is due to moulding and an accumulation of fluid on the tip of the baby's head (the caput). Don't worry—your baby's head will return to its normal shape within a day or so. It is designed to be soft so that it can mould to an appropriate shape during its passage through the birth canal.

Vacuum

In a vacuum delivery, your doctor places a plastic or metal cup against your baby's head and a vacuum is then created by suction. The doctor pulls in concert with your contractions and pushing until the baby's head is delivered. An episiotomy is almost inevitable with either forceps or vacuum delivery. After delivery, your baby will probably have a swelling on the scalp where the cup was applied and the vacuum created. The swelling will subside over the next few days.

Forceps

Forceps are metal instruments shaped like large, curved spoons with hollow heads. They are placed on either side of the baby's head and the doctor pulls on them as the mother pushes during a contraction. The amount of force required varies enormously depending on how large the baby is, how far down the pelvis the baby is, how strong contractions are and how effective the mother's pushing is.

Your baby will usually, though not always, have some pressure markings on his or her head from the forceps after delivery but these marks fade rapidly. They are similar to the impressions left on your own skin when you sleep on a fold of clothing. Occasionally there may be some bruising or other marking from the forceps but this too will probably fade within days of delivery.

Rotational forceps

Rotational forceps are rarely used nowadays and have been abandoned completely in some hospitals (they have largely been replaced by the vacuum). They are used when the baby's head has not rotated spontaneously into the normal position for birth (occipito anterior or face down). These forceps are associated with an increased risk of trauma to both mother and baby.

Recovery from assisted delivery may be slower than from normal, spontaneous vaginal delivery. The slower recovery may be because your labour was long and you are exhausted or because you have a larger episiotomy than you would have had with a normal birth.

Induction

Induction of labour is the process of artificially starting labour before it begins spontaneously. Often, induction is confused with acceleration of labour that has already begun spontaneously. This form of medical intervention may seem very attractive if you are overdue or finding it hard going at the end of your pregnancy. You may wish to get it all over with and actually see your baby. This is very natural but you shouldn't set your heart on it.

Most women go into labour within a few days either side of their due date which falls 40 weeks after the last menstrual period. However, with a first baby, it is not at all unusual to go a week to 10 days past the due date. In general, your best chance at having a normal labour and birth is if you go into labour yourself without having your labour started artificially. Obviously, the longer you go over, the more likely it is you'll become anxious and fed up.

If you go more than 10–12 days overdue, in most cases you will have either a scan to assess the amount of fluid around the baby or an internal exam to see if your cervix is favourable (soft and shortened) for induction. Whether your labour is induced or not will depend on a variety of factors, including how well you are coping with being overdue, the condition of your cervix, the results of your scan and the attitude of your doctor. Most doctors would prefer to induce labour if you are 2 weeks overdue. This is because there is a risk that the placenta may not continue to function as efficiently as it has done during the rest of your pregnancy and this can place your baby at risk of lack of oxygen.

If induction were a simple procedure that always worked it would be easy to make a decision about whether or not to be induced. Unfortunately, induction doesn't always work and starting the process may precipitate a cascade of problems that wouldn't have occurred if labour started spontaneously. Depending on the circumstances, labour may be longer, more painful, the baby may be more stressed and you may end up either with an assisted vaginal delivery (vacuum or forceps), or caesarean section, which would not have been necessary if your labour had started itself.

Of course, induction can often be very successful and result in a normal labour and normal delivery. A successful outcome is more likely if you have given birth vaginally before and if your cervix is 'favourable'. If it is your first baby, the process is likely to be more difficult and complicated.

If you are keen to be induced, discuss it with your doctor. In general, it is not advisable to induce labour for non-medical reasons. You should try and take the long view and strike a balance between your enthusiasm for getting the baby delivered and the risks of induction.

Reasons for induction

The most common reason for induction is because a pregnancy has gone past its due date. Because you have a better chance of having a normal labour and delivery if nature takes its course and labour starts on its own, most women, and doctors, are reluctant to attempt to induce labour until at least 10 days after the EDD. Most doctors advise putting a limit of 14 days past the EDD and would prefer to induce labour at that point. It is important to clarify your due dates early in pregnancy so that if you go past your EDD everyone knows where they stand.

You are more likely to go overdue on your first pregnancy, but if you go overdue on subsequent pregnancies, induction is usually a straightforward process.

The amount of amniotic fluid around your baby may diminish if you go significantly overdue and may be the ultimate reason for induction.

After 'post-dates', the most frequent reasons for induction include:

- False labour (contractions without the other signs of labour, e.g. dilatation of the cervix)
- Spontaneous rupture of the membranes (breaking of the waters) before labour
- High blood pressure/pre-eclampsia
- Suspicion the baby may not be growing properly
- Bleeding in late pregnancy
- Twins.

Other uncommon conditions like diabetes or a previous history of stillbirth may also lead to induction. Social reasons are also fairly common, especially on second and subsequent births. These may include travel plans, availability of help at home, work commitments and distance from hospital.

Methods of induction

Artificial rupture of the membranes (ARM)

ARM, or breaking of the waters, is the most common method of induction, especially when the cervix is favourable (soft and shortened). In some hospitals, oxytocin is given intravenously very soon afterwards; in others there is a delay overnight in the expectation that you will start labour yourself in a more natural way. The disadvantage of giving oxytocin early is that you will have pains or contractions with it; whereas if you wait overnight you will have a 70–80 per cent chance of starting labour yourself and may never need oxytocin at all. If it is not your first birth you have more than a 90 per cent chance of starting labour with ARM alone. The favourability of your cervix will determine to a large extent the success of ARM alone.

You will have a vaginal examination to assess the favourability of your cervix prior to induction no matter what method of induction is chosen. Some doctors use a scoring system, the Bishop score, to describe the cervix, taking into account the length, consistency and elasticity of the cervix as well as the position of the baby's head in the pelvis. You may see a reference to the Bishop score in your chart.

ARM involves a vaginal examination during which your waters are broken by a hook (amnihook) or with forceps. From your point of view there is no difference. This can be an uncomfortable experience as it can take a few attempts to puncture the membranes. Amniotic fluid will begin to drain immediately—initially in large gushes and then more slowly. Sometimes very little fluid drains because the fluid may be behind the baby's head or because there is very little left. You may be given a sample of the fluid in a test tube to keep with you until transfer to the labour ward.

Oxytocin

Oxytocin will almost always cause contractions in a pregnant woman, but artificially induced contractions may not signify that labour is starting and that the induction is going to be successful. Remember, there is more to labour than contractions of the uterus. Your cervix must also dilate for labour to commence. After an oxytocin infusion has started you should have a good indication within 6 hours at most as to whether or not the induction is going to work. Your labour may start but not progress and you may require a caesarean section. This scenario, 'arrest of progress', is more frequent with inductions and is one of the reasons why induction should not be undertaken lightly.

Prostaglandins

Prostaglandins are also frequently used to induce labour. This group of chemicals are also found naturally in the body (in semen) and are closely involved in the reproductive system. Artificially produced prostaglandin, when inserted into the vagina close to the cervix, causes the cervix to soften and may initiate uterine contractions. The response to prostaglandins is quite variable from woman to woman and depends on a number of factors—the favourability of the cervix, the stage of pregnancy, and whether it is a first pregnancy. Some women experience strong contractions, 'prostin pains', but labour does not start immediately and this can be frustrating. Rarely, prostaglandins cause extremely strong contractions that can be dangerous for the baby, and sometimes even for the mother. This is, thankfully, unusual. Sometimes prostaglandin insertion is followed by contractions that subside and then the waters break spontaneously. This may precede spontaneous labour or oxytocin may be required to induce labour. Prostaglandins are most frequently used in post-dates pregnancies and when the cervix is not favourable for ARM.

Frequently asked questions

Is induced labour more painful?
Yes, if oxytocin is used the contractions can be more intense.

How overdue will I be allowed to go before I must be induced?
Most doctors advise an upper limit of 42 weeks and are uncomfortable with a pregnancy going beyond 14 days overdue. If there is uncertainty about your dates, however, there may be room for deferring induction.

If I have stitches will they have to be taken out?
No. Stitches nowadays are dissolvable.

I have a friend who had to have her stitches redone a few months after her baby was born. Is this common?
No. Sometimes the perineum can heal in a way that makes intercourse painful. If this happens it may be necessary to perform a small operation to refashion the perineum.

I didn't have stitches the first time. Am I less likely to need them the second time round?
It would be most unusual to have stitches after a second birth if you didn't need them the first time.

Should I save cord blood in case my baby needs stem cell treatment at some time in the future?
"No" is the simple answer. There are a few extremely rare conditions for which cord blood stem cell treatment is currently available and it is best to use blood that is not from the affected individual. If your child should need treatment in the future, cord blood stem cells will be collected from another donor. Collection and storage is available commercially, is very expensive, and is not facilitated in Irish hospitals as it is not clinically indicated, except in exceptional circumstances when it will be done for you.

8 caesarean section

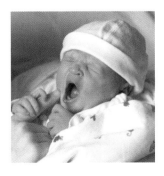

If your doctor tells you that your baby is going to have to be delivered by caesarean section, don't panic. As an operation, caesarean section is now a very common, safe and painless procedure, due to improvements in anaesthesia, blood transfusion services and antibiotics. Your baby will be delivered through an incision across the bottom of your abdomen on your panty line. It is usually done under spinal anaesthetic, you can be awake for the birth, your partner can be present and you should make a quick recovery.

Increased frequency of caesarean sections

Caesarean section has increased in frequency throughout the Western world and Ireland is no exception to this trend. In the 1970s fewer than 10 per cent of babies were delivered by section, whereas now the figure is greater than 20 per cent. The rate varies from one hospital to another and is more common on a first pregnancy.

There are many reasons for the increase in caesarean births. The primary medical reasons are related to the way first labours are managed in hospital and more continuous monitoring of the baby's heart rate in labour. There are of course other reasons apart from these for the increase in caesareans. For example, it is now common practice for breech babies to be delivered by caesarean section. Also, women who have had one previous caesarean after an unhappy first labour experience are more likely to request another caesarean, and doctors are more likely to accede to their requests. Finally, many very premature babies are now delivered by caesarean to minimise trauma to them—because of huge improvements in neonatal intensive care, they have a better chance than ever of surviving.

The increase in caesareans has also, sadly, been influenced by litigation. Doctors know they are much less likely to be sued successfully if they have delivered a baby by caesarean section and this exerts a subtle pressure on their decision-making.

Elective and emergency caesareans

Caesareans may be either emergency or elective. All caesareans performed during labour are described medically as emergencies, whereas caesareans before labour may be either 'elective' or emergency procedures.

The two most common reasons for caesarean section during labour are arrest of progress, and suspected foetal distress. Both are far more common in first labours. Arrest of progress may also be described as failure to progress, failure to dilate, or dystocia.

Emergency sections before labour are frequently performed because of bleeding from a separating placenta, severe pre-eclampsia that is deteriorating rapidly, or suspected foetal distress.

Elective caesareans are when you are given a date in advance and you come into the hospital for a planned delivery. Common indications for electives are repeat operations (if you have had two previous sections), breech presentation, and serious problems on a previous pregnancy like damage to the rectum. If you are having twins and the first is breech, you are more likely to have a caesarean, although twin pregnancy of itself is not usually an indication for caesarean section.

Caesarean on request

If for some reason you want to have a caesarean section, you will have to convince your doctor to perform one. Sometimes women who have had a very difficult first birth ask for one, even though second births are generally easier. Bring up the topic early in your pregnancy and discuss the pros and cons of the operation. Potentially, caesarean birth is more complicated than normal because it increases the chances of your needing a blood transfusion and of getting an infection or a clot in your leg. Another disadvantage is that it usually takes longer to recover from a section and sections may have implications for your future health. It may influence how your babies are delivered in the future and may have an impact on gynaecological surgery you may need later in life. For these reasons, if you have a choice, vaginal delivery is your best option.

The process of caesarean section

The majority of caesareans are performed under spinal anaesthesia, which is similar to an epidural, but faster to take effect and deeper. General anaesthesia is not commonly used these days. The final decision about the type of anaesthesia used rests with the anaesthetist who will make the decision based on safety reasons. Under spinal anaesthesia, you are awake and usually your partner can be present for the actual birth. A complete pubic shave is unnecessary but you will probably be given a trim. After the spinal has been inserted, the lower half of your body will go numb quite rapidly and when the anaesthetist is satisfied with the level of pain relief achieved, the operation commences.

tubal ligation

If you decide well before the section is performed that your family is complete and you do not wish to become pregnant again, a tubal ligation (the tying of the fallopian tubes) can be performed after the caesarean delivery. Medically, it is an ideal time to perform the operation as it will save you a subsequent operation, but any decision to take this route must be well thought out beforehand. The procedure will not be performed on the spur of the moment.

If it is performed at the time of your caesarean section, the operation will take an extra ten minutes or so. A small section of each fallopian tube or the whole tube is removed and the blind end tied off. Tubal ligation has no effect whatsoever on your recovery from caesarean section.

Your bladder will be emptied by the surgeon or assistant and your abdomen will be painted with an antiseptic to minimise the risk of infection. Next, a sterile drape will be placed over your abdomen and legs and draped over a support rail over your chest. The surgeon will test that your level of pain relief is adequate (and if it is you won't be aware of this) and then the operation will begin. At this stage your partner, wearing a gown, a hat, and possibly a mask, will be brought to your side. He will be put sitting with his back to the operation, facing your head. You will feel some pressure and perhaps a pulling sensation but you should feel no pain whatsoever.

In a very small proportion of cases (less than 1 per cent) the spinal will take either incompletely or not at all. If this happens you will need to have a general anaesthetic.

It usually takes no more than 10–15 minutes from the time the spinal takes effect for your baby to be born, while the rest of the operation may take another 10–15 minutes. You generally won't be able to see any of the actual surgery because of the drape over your chest. Even if you could see it would seem as though it were happening to someone else because of the anaesthetic.

At the moment the baby is actually delivered you may feel additional pressure on your upper abdomen as the baby is pushed down by the surgeon's assistant. The obstetrician performing the operation will show you the baby and then hand him or her over to the attending paediatrician. Your baby will be checked briefly and may be weighed in the operating theatre. The baby will be wrapped to prevent heat loss and given to your partner sitting at your side. Because your movement is restricted it may be difficult for you to touch the baby immediately but you should be able to at least give him or her a kiss! It will also be difficult for you to breastfeed at this stage.

While you are distracted by the baby, the obstetrician completes the operation and you will be surprised by how quickly it is over with. You should request dissolving stitches in your skin so that you will not have to have stitches removed later. Your baby will go to the post-natal ward and you will be transferred to a recovery area for an hour or so until you have feeling back in your legs and your doctors are satisfied that your condition is stable. You will then be transferred to the post-natal ward to be reunited with your baby.

After a caesarean

Recovery from caesarean section depends on many factors, among the most important are your attitude and happiness with the procedure. Your recovery is likely to be quicker if you have an epidural or spinal anaesthetic rather than a general. The circumstances

types of incision

Virtually all caesareans are now performed through a horizontal incision in the lower part of the uterus. The cut in the skin is usually along the bikini line. The scar on your abdomen does not indicate what sort of scar is on your uterus. In the distant past, most caesareans were done via a vertical incision in the uterus, a 'classical' caesarean section. This scar was associated with a high risk of rupture in a subsequent pregnancy and is now only performed in very rare circumstances indeed.

surrounding your section will also affect your recovery. An emergency caesarean performed after you have been in labour for several hours, perhaps following induction of labour and when you had been anticipating a normal vaginal delivery, will be more difficult to recover from than an elective caesarean that you planned for and were happy with.

If you are at all unclear about the reasons for your caesarean you should discuss this with your doctor. You may wish to wait until your six week check-up and this will give you time to get your thoughts in order. Let your obstetrician know in advance if you wish to discuss your labour/delivery so that the hospital records can be available for review.

Some women who have caesareans feel they have missed out on something by not having given birth vaginally. This reaction has to be balanced against the reality that there were good reasons for having the caesarean in the first place. Also, it should be borne in mind that the vast majority of women—80 per cent—who have caesareans are able to give birth vaginally subsequently.

Normally, you will be fit for discharge home within five to seven days if the operation has been uncomplicated and there have been no problems immediately before or after delivery. You may require iron tablets for a few weeks after a caesarean, and rarely a blood transfusion may be required (because the blood loss at caesarean delivery is usually more than at a vaginal delivery).

Catheter

If the section was performed after you went into labour you will probably have a catheter in place for a day or so, whereas this is less likely with an elective section.

Pain relief

Pain relief is usually given intravenously for the first 24 hours and may be in a form you control yourself, 'patient controlled analgesia' or PCA. Morphine is the usual drug given this way. A pump mechanism is connected to your drip and you press a button whenever you need more pain relief. There is a locking mechanism in the device to prevent you from giving yourself an overdose. Morphine may make you nauseated and some women develop an itch from it. After the first 24 hours you will probably get pain relievers in either tablet or suppository form.

a mother's tips

Take it easy. Don't expect to jump up out of your hospital bed the day after the operation. Take things slowly and use small steps to get around at first.

Take your pain relief. Even if you are breastfeeding, the amount of medication that will go through into your milk is negligible.

Accept help. If family and friends offer to lend a hand with errands, chores etc, accept their help graciously.

Avoid stairs. At least for the first week you are home, make a base downstairs.

Sit up carefully. Either pull yourself into a sitting position from lying down by getting leverage off your furniture or get someone to help you. When you get out of bed, roll off on to one knee then stand gently, pulling yourself up by using a chair.

Avoid fatty foods and fizzy drinks. Once your bowels start to work properly again you may find you are very windy.

Keep necessities close by. Fill a basket with all the baby supplies you need, your pain medication, etc. and keep it close at hand so you don't have to constantly fetch things. Keep a pillow close by. If you find it painful to laugh, sneeze or cough, press a soft pillow to your tummy gently.

The form of pain relief given may depend on whether you are breastfeeding or not. Most pain relievers are safe when breastfeeding and indeed a trace of morphine in your system may do less harm than surges of adrenalin from coping with pain.

Breastfeeding

You will probably have your first chance to breastfeed your baby within two hours of delivery. It shouldn't be more difficult to do so than if you had had a vaginal delivery, although you may find it easier to use certain positions than others. The midwife can show you ways to prop your baby, perhaps on a pile of pillows, to keep pressure off your wound.

Preventing clots

The day after the caesarean you will be helped out of bed and encouraged to walk. This is to help your recovery and reduce the chance of a clot forming in your veins. You will also be given anti-clot medication to further reduce the risk. The physiotherapy staff will show you which exercises will best assist your recovery.

Wound healing

The wound in your abdomen is usually across the lower part just at the hairline or below it. If the stitches in your skin are dissolving they will not require removal. Some stitches do need removal and this will be done prior to going home. After you go home you may find your wound painful as you get into more active daily activities like lifting your baby. A silk scarf placed between your skin and clothing may ease the pain and discomfort. You should set your own pace in terms of activities, with the limiting factor being pain. You will probably be comfortable enough to drive within three to four weeks but bring another driver with you so that if you find it too painful, your companion can take over. Also, check with your insurance company to make sure you are covered.

Afterpains

Afterpains following a caesarean may be more painful because of the scar on your uterus but you should have adequate pain relief. You may find that emptying your bladder is also a little uncomfortable or painful for a few weeks after a caesarean. This is because the bladder is close to the scar on your uterus and it may stretch your internal scar, particularly at the end of passing water.

Exercise

It is not a good idea to start specific exercises before your six-week check, other than walking, but swimming is fine if you feel up to it. After your six-week check, you will probably be interested in exercises targeted at your tummy. Sit-ups alone will not tone the area. You will need to do aerobic exercise as well if you want to see any outward improvement in your shape. Start aerobic exercise gently and build up your stamina gradually.

Future implications

Caesarean section leaves you with a scar on both your abdomen and uterus and this may have implications for you in the long term. If you have another baby for example, you are more likely to require another caesarean (although 70–80 per cent of subsequent births are vaginal) and the risk of complications such as haemorrhage are increased. If you require a hysterectomy at some stage, the presence of scar tissue may make the procedure more complicated or prevent you from having a vaginal hysterectomy as opposed to an abdominal one.

possible complications of caesarean sections

Haemorrhage

You can expect to lose more blood if your baby is born by caesarean section. Sometimes the amount of blood lost requires a blood transfusion. Your risk of this is less than 10 per cent unless you have placenta praevia or were haemorrhaging before the section.

Wound infection

You will have a scar on your abdomen after a section and this can sometimes get infected. The risk is low and you will be given antibiotics during the operation in order to reduce the risk further. An infection shows in an area of redness, which is hot, around the scar. There may be a swelling and possibly a discharge from the scar. Your temperature may be raised.

Clots in the legs

This is a rare complication but is more common after a caesarean section than after vaginal delivery. There is a remote risk that a clot could detach itself, travel to your lungs and be fatal. Getting up and about soon after any surgery reduces the risk. You may also be prescribed injections to help prevent clot formation.

Hysterectomy

The risk of needing a hysterectomy at the time of a caesarean section is very low, less than 1 in 1000. It is more likely if you have had a previous caesarean, especially if the placenta is low and under your previous scar. While this complication is quite rare, it is a real risk and is one of the reasons you should think long and hard before electing to have a medically unnecessary caesarean.

Frequently asked questions

I had my last baby by caesarean section. Am I going to be able to have a normal delivery this time?
You will have an approximately 80 per cent chance of a vaginal delivery depending on the reason for your last section and the way the baby is lying.

How many sections is it safe to have?
As many as you want but each naturally has a risk (transfusion, infection etc.) that increases with each successive operation.

How big will my scar be?
About 10 cm (6 inches) long.

If I have another section will my scar be in the same place?
Yes, usually. Repeated incisions through the same scar do tend to heal more slowly, however.

Is post-natal depression more common with caesareans?
No is the simple answer, but it does depend on the circumstances surrounding your delivery. For example, if you were very disappointed about not having a normal birth it is more likely you will get depressed.

The spinal didn't take last time and I needed a general anaesthetic. Is the same thing likely to happen again?
No, it is extremely unusual for a spinal not to work twice unless there is some abnormality of your spine that you were unaware of. If you are concerned you can ask to be reviewed before your section by an anaesthetist to discuss pain relief for a future delivery (caesarean or vaginal).

It's been a year since my section and I still feel twinges in my scar. Is that normal?
No, your scar should be virtually forgotten at that stage. If you are concerned discuss it with your GP in the first instance.

How long do I have to wait before another pregnancy?
As soon as your periods return you are fertile again and may become pregnant any time thereafter. Your body is ready as soon as you start your periods. Even if you were to get pregnant within three or four months it would be a year from your caesarean before you were ready to give birth again.

Is my child more likely to develop autism if I have a caesarean section?
No, caesarean delivery does not increase the likelihood of developing autism.

9 twins and triplets

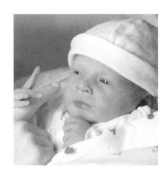

Having one baby, particularly your first, is one of the most emotionally charged events in life, so having two (or more!) at the same time is quite an extra challenge. You may have very mixed emotions about it. Delight and excitement may be tempered with fear about how you will manage, especially if you already have children. If you planned to have one more child to complete your family and are now faced with the prospect of two, you may feel overwhelmed. These feelings are quite natural.

Twins

There are two types of twins, identical and non-identical, or fraternal. Identical twins are also known medically as monozygotic (from one zygote or fertilised egg), while non-identical twins are dizygotic, arising from two separate eggs. Identical twins occur because a single fertilised egg splits in two. They are examples of cloning in nature.

rates of twin pregnancy

The frequency of twin pregnancy in Ireland is approximately 1–2 per cent. Most of these are non-identical twins. Some countries have higher rates of non-identical twin births; they are four times more common in Africa than in China, for example. The highest rate is in the Yoruba people from Nigeria.

Non-identical or fraternal twins are created when a woman just happens to get pregnant twice at the same time because she has released two eggs and both have been fertilised. If you are a fraternal twin yourself, your chances of having twins increases almost five-fold.

Identical twins are normally formed very soon after fertilisation. If division occurs very early, there are two separate placentas and separate sacs in which the twins develop. If there is a delay in splitting into two there is an increased chance of complications. The most extreme example of delayed division is conjoined, or Siamese, twins. Siamese twins are extremely rare and can be seen clearly on ultrasound scan. The more usual effect of slightly delayed division is a common, shared, placenta and this may give rise to serious complications as a result of shared blood circulation.

Early in your pregnancy a scan will be performed to try and determine if your twins are identical or not. If they are not, you can relax. If your twins are thought to be identical, you will be followed more closely to try and detect problems early.

Diagnosing twin pregnancy

Women who are carrying twins usually, although not always, have more pronounced pregnancy symptoms such as vomiting in early pregnancy. Your doctor may be suspicious of a twin pregnancy if your uterus is larger than expected for the period of pregnancy (large for dates). The suspicion will either be confirmed or quashed after you have an ultrasound scan. In any case, most women with severe vomiting do not have twins. At the time of diagnosis an effort, usually successful, will be made to determine if the twins are identical or not.

A significant number of very early diagnosed twin pregnancies finish as single pregnancies. This is because there is a high mortality rate among twins early in pregnancy. There may be no sign, such as bleeding, that one of the embryos has died; the only evidence may be a small second sac seen on ultrasound. Generally this does not cause any problems to the surviving twin and after the birth there may be nothing at all to indicate that a second embryo was present earlier on. Sometimes the loss of one twin in early pregnancy may reveal itself by some bleeding (threatened abortion) and a scan will reveal a small, perhaps collapsed, second sac. The loss of one twin very early in pregnancy, in the first 10 or 12 weeks, rarely causes any problems.

Complications

Although there are increased risks of complications in a twin pregnancy, most result in the safe delivery of two healthy children. The main risks are a greater chance of premature delivery and caesarean section.

Pre-eclampsia and diabetes are more common in women carrying twins. These complications occur most often in the third trimester, or last three months, so your pregnancy will be monitored more closely from 28 weeks onwards. Premature labour, although more frequent than with a single pregnancy, is still uncommon. Most twins deliver soon after 37 weeks (as opposed to the usual 40 weeks) but a small proportion deliver sooner. The chances of survival increase dramatically from 26 weeks onwards.

An identical twin may die suddenly at any stage of pregnancy, but this is a very rare occurrence with fraternal twins.

Twin transfusion syndrome

One of the most frequent causes of death in identical twin pregnancy is twin transfusion syndrome. It may occur at any stage, even in labour. It is the main complication looked for in the antenatal care of a twin pregnancy. If the condition develops slowly there is usually a major difference in size between the twins and there is excess fluid in one of the sacs. This will be diagnosed on ultrasound and is one reason for following a twin pregnancy with regular scans from about 28 weeks onwards.

Twin transfusion syndrome may cause the death of one twin either gradually or as a sudden event and will put the survivor at an increased risk of brain damage. Although uncommon, the condition is extremely difficult to deal with. Laser treatment to block the communicating blood vessels is available in specialised foetal medicine departments.

Rachel's twins

Rachel didn't find out she was having twins until she was 25 weeks pregnant. 'Since it was my first pregnancy I had nothing to compare it to so when I had morning sickness I didn't know if it was any worse than normal. I have quite a small build too so even though I felt enormous I wasn't and so my doctor didn't suspect I was having twins. When I finally had a routine ultrasound and she told me about the babies, I was really thrown. I couldn't believe I was so out of touch with what was going on inside me that I hadn't even suspected there were two babies. Mentally, I didn't recover from the shock until well after the girls were born.'

It is a complicated procedure and carries with it the risk of premature delivery. If you show signs of developing twin transfusion syndrome you will be referred by your consultant for consideration for laser treatment. There is nothing you can do yourself to prevent twin transfusion syndrome from developing.

Congenital malformation

Another cause of death in twin pregnancy is congenital malformation, which is twice as likely to occur in a twin pregnancy. The background risk of a major congenital malformation is approximately 2 per cent so in a twin pregnancy, it is 4 per cent. Remember, this means there is a 96 per cent chance all will be well.

Prematurity

Premature birth is much more common with multiple pregnancies. The lower limit of survival age is 24 weeks gestation. The chances of survival at this stage are very slim, however, and among survivors the risk of disability is significant. From 28 weeks onwards the chances of survival increase dramatically and the risk of disability diminishes progressively.

Premature birth is more common with multiple pregnancies because labour starts spontaneously or because there is a complication requiring delivery such as pre-eclampsia or bleeding. The most common problem associated with premature labour is accumulation of excessive amniotic fluid in identical twin pregnancies. The excess fluid expands the uterus significantly and causes labour to start. In practice this is only a danger in identical twin pregnancy.

Special considerations

If you are working outside the home, be sure to allow yourself more rest with a twin pregnancy. You will inevitably be more tired and uncomfortable earlier than you would be in a single pregnancy. It is hard to predict just how soon you will run out of steam but it would be safe to anticipate that you will be pretty tired by 34 weeks. If you can lighten your workload, try to do so to avoid getting run down. If you are planning to travel, you may find flying very uncomfortable after 28 weeks.

Unfortunately, you are not legally entitled to any extra leave or financial help with twins—entitlements only increase if you have triplets.

---

when a twin dies

The death of one twin, and survival of the other, is a particularly distressing event for any couple. Thankfully, this is a rare event, occurring in less than 10 per cent of twin pregnancies. You will be faced with contrasting emotions of grief at the death of one baby and happiness at the birth of the other. Dealing with these conflicting emotions while undergoing intense hormonal changes will be extremely difficult and may require special counselling, which should be available through most hospitals.

Delivery of twins

The method of delivery, caesarean or vaginal, will be determined to a large extent by which way your first baby is lying. If the head is presenting first, the usual way, you have a very good chance of a normal vaginal delivery. If your first twin is presenting breech, or bottom first, your chances of caesarean delivery are significantly increased. The decision about method of delivery is best discussed with your obstetrician late in the pregnancy. Because twins are usually smaller than single babies, because of competition for nutrition and being born sooner, the actual delivery process may be physically easier for you.

After your first twin is delivered, the obstetrician will determine which way your second baby is lying, either by examining your abdomen or by using an ultrasound scanner in the delivery ward. If the second baby is coming head first you can expect a normal delivery. The doctor will break the waters of the second twin if they have not broken already and you will then push with each contraction as for your first. The interval between a first and second twin averages 15 minutes but the interval may be much shorter or extend to a few hours.

If your second baby is presenting as a breech, the doctor may either turn the baby to head first or may decide to proceed with a vaginal breech delivery. From your point of view the procedure is broadly similar: your waters are broken and then you push with each contraction! From the doctor's point of view, a vaginal breech delivery is slightly more complicated as it involves more manipulation and skill than a normal, head-first delivery. The least-preferable situation is a vaginal first delivery followed by a caesarean for the second twin. Thankfully, this is not very common.

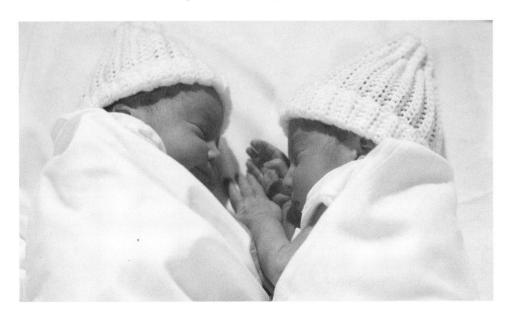

The third stage of labour, delivery of the placentas, is the same as with a single baby delivery. After delivery of the second twin you will be given an injection to assist contraction of the uterus and separation of the placentas and to control bleeding. The placentas will be delivered together. Frequently they are joined together, particularly if the twins are identical.

Breastfeeding

There is no reason why you shouldn't be able to breastfeed. Obviously, you will need more help in the early days, especially if this is your first pregnancy. If you have already breastfed you will find it easier. The midwives in hospital will help you find the most comfortable positions and establish a timetable so you can try to get a break from feeding now and then. You needn't worry about not producing enough milk for two babies—as long as you continue to feed them, your body will produce enough milk for them. There is no guarantee however that the babies will be hungry at the same times so feeding sessions may last so long they seem to merge into each other—but this is the case whether you choose breast or bottle. Some parents find that they can successfully combine breast and bottle feeding so that the mother gets some relief from feeding demands if she needs it.

How will I manage?

Most parents of twins worry during the course of the pregnancy about how they are going to cope with the demands of two babies. In the hours and days immediately

two for the price of one

When Brian and Marie, in their mid-thirties, found out they were having twin boys, they were thrilled. Then panic set in. As Brian remembers:

'Of course, we didn't know what to expect but I was thrilled that we were getting a jumpstart to our family since we started a bit late. Two for the price of one. I thought the best approach was just to try and not do too much except look after the babies and to be there as a second pair of hands for my wife whenever I could. I was more worried about her than anything—I thought she'd be exhausted and since neither of us had any experience of little babies I knew she was really worried about how to do things right. For the first few weeks we didn't get much sleep it has to be said—if the twins were asleep we were too wired to sleep ourselves. We got over that quickly though and started sleeping through some of their more minor restlessness. In fact, we found that when they were asleep together in the Moses basket they sort of comforted each other. Feeding was the biggest challenge—we fed them at the same time—if one of them was hungry Marie would take them and a few minutes later I'd just automatically give the other one a bottle until they were more or less in synch. When I was at work, Marie's sister or mum would fill in. That lasted for a few weeks and by then we had more confidence and could manage solo. For about a year though, when we needed to see people socially we'd have them around for a takeaway and they'd usually end up helping out a bit too. It sounds like a dreadful cliché but you just have to take it a day at a time and before you know it, things settle down a bit.'

following the birth, these anxieties and normal post-natal hormones may make an overwhelming combination. There is no doubt that caring for two infants of the same age tests most people's stamina, but people do manage, one way or another.

Triplets and quadruplets

Most multiple births are twins. Higher order births—triplets and upwards—are much less common but are more likely if you have taken fertility treatments. Triplets usually consist of one set of identical twins and a third baby. In other words, twins are conceived but one of the twin embryos splits to form a set of identical twins. With an IVF pregnancy, or one conceived following fertility treatment, three separate eggs may have been fertilised. Nowadays, following IVF treatment it is standard practice to put no more than one or two embryos in the uterus.

Complications

The main complication that makes a triplet pregnancy different from a twin pregnancy is prematurity. It is unusual for a triple pregnancy to last longer than 34 weeks. Your chances of caesarean section are also significantly increased, partly because of prematurity but mainly because most obstetricians are uncomfortable delivering triplets vaginally.

Apart from prematurity and increased chance of caesarean, the other main difference with a triplet pregnancy is that the symptoms of pregnancy are more pronounced. This is the case with quadruplet pregnancy, too. Obviously, quadruplet pregnancies are very rare—the National Maternity Hospital might see one case every three to four years. The very thought is daunting and physically, the challenge of carrying four babies is tremendous. In a quad pregnancy, the risk of prematurity increases and caesarean section becomes much more likely. In fact, caesarean section is the norm with quads. If you are carrying quads, you are bound to be very uncomfortable from the combined weight of four babies, their placentas and amniotic fluid and you must take extra care not to wear yourself out. It is unusual for a quadruplet pregnancy to progress beyond 32 weeks and many will deliver too prematurely for the babies to survive.

With a multiple pregnancy, there is a greater than normal chance of your baby requiring admission to the special care baby unit, primarily because of prematurity. This is almost inevitable if your babies are born at 34 weeks or less, as most triplets, and virtually all quads are. After 34 weeks, the chances of your babies requiring admission to the baby unit diminish progressively so that by 36–37 weeks it is unusual for them to need admission. Sometimes twins are dramatically different in size and if one is very small, usually less than 2.2 kg (4 lb), the paediatricians will recommend admission for a period of observation to ensure that feeding is established well and to prevent the baby from having low blood sugar levels.

Breastfeeding

Breastfeeding is still possible if your babies are admitted to special care but is obviously more challenging logistically. If you can, try to feed your babies yourself—breast milk provides the optimum nutrition for all newborns and is especially important to more vulnerable babies. The midwives will do their best to help you with feeding. If your babies are unable to feed at your breast, you can express milk so they can be fed it by bottle or tube.

Frequently asked questions

I am pregnant with twins. Should I take extra folic acid supplements?
Yes, you should double the dosage to 600 mg a day.

I am daunted by the idea of breastfeeding twins. Who can help me try?
Your midwife will advise and assist you and if you wish will also put you in touch with Cuidiú—the Irish Childbirth Trust (www.cuidiu-ict.ie) or La Lèche League (www.lalecheleagueireland.com). The League offers special advice and has regular meetings throughout the country.

Is it advisable to extend my maternity leave?
Yes. Take more time off before delivery and after if you can. Expect delivery no later than 38 weeks with twins and 34 weeks with triplets—so plan to stop at 35 weeks and 30 weeks respectively.

Is it possible to be pregnant with twins and not find out until delivery?
Yes, although it is very unusual nowadays because most women have had at least one scan during pregnancy and it would be very unusual to miss a twin pregnancy.

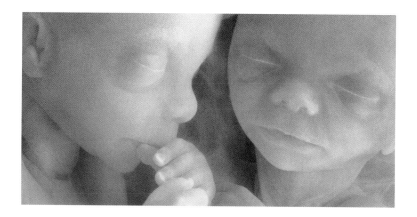

10 infertility

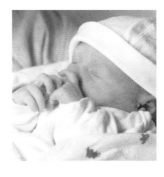

Don't expect to get pregnant immediately you start trying. It is perfectly normal to take up to a year to conceive even when having regular intercourse during the fertile period. Statistically, you have an 80 per cent chance of getting pregnant in the first year of trying and a 90 per cent chance of conceiving within two years if there are no underlying problems. You should therefore give it a year before you start becoming concerned about infertility problems. (If you are very anxious before this year is up, by all means ask your GP for advice.)

If you do have trouble getting pregnant, you are not alone. The good news is that there are now more support mechanisms and medical options in place for you than ever before. The best care will attempt to address both your medical and your emotional needs.

Primary and secondary infertility

Infertility is medically defined as failure to achieve a pregnancy within one year of trying. If you have never been pregnant before and are having trouble getting pregnant you will be treated for primary infertility.

If you have been pregnant before, regardless of how that pregnancy ended, you will be treated for secondary infertility. This occurs when a woman has been pregnant before but experiences difficulty conceiving after that pregnancy. Because a woman's ability to get pregnant diminishes with advancing age, secondary infertility is even more common than primary infertility. If you already have a child secondary infertility is not treated as sympathetically by society and can be a source of tremendous distress. If you had problems conceiving your first child, the cause of secondary infertility may be the same and hopefully can be dealt with in the same way that met with success the first time. If you did not have trouble the first time, you may have taken for granted that you would be able to have another baby relatively easily; it may take you longer to seek help if this is the case.

Unless your partner has had a major illness it is unlikely that there has been a substantial reduction in the quantity or quality of his sperm so investigations will probably focus on you. On the other hand, if you have a new partner he should have himself checked, even if he has already fathered children with another woman. Otherwise, the principles of investigation and appropriate treatments are the same whether infertility is primary or secondary.

Infertility may be caused by a number of problems involving the woman, the man or both but in approximately 10 per cent of cases the cause remains a mystery. Up to one-third of couples with unexplained infertility will eventually achieve a successful pregnancy without treatment. However, if this has not happened in four years of trying, the likelihood of unassisted pregnancy is very small.

If you have no fertility problems as a couple, you have a 60 per cent chance of becoming pregnant within six months of starting to try, and a 90 per cent chance of success within two years.

The complex process of fertilisation

Although the specific details of fertilisation of an egg by a sperm are well understood, and reproducible in a laboratory to some extent, what makes any given encounter between a healthy sperm and a healthy egg a fertile one is less well understood. This is one of the more frustrating aspects of infertility.

Each month, in the middle of your cycle, one or two eggs are ejected from one of your ovaries (where they have been since before you were born). The average woman produces about twelve eggs each year. If you started to ovulate and have periods at the age of 11, by the time you are 30 you will have expelled 228 eggs, all of which were theoretically capable of being fertilised. If you have been taking the oral contraceptive pill, however, you have effectively been 'saving' your eggs because your ovulation has been suppressed while you took the pill. So, taking the pill may actually work to your advantage in the long term when it comes to fertility! There is no scientific evidence to support this, although it's a nice thought. There is no evidence that taking the pill reduces your fertility.

Once you have ovulated, the egg needs to fuse with a sperm in order for you to get pregnant. The process of fertilisation is extremely complex so it is no wonder it is fraught with potential setbacks.

With each act of intercourse, between 200 and 300 million sperm are deposited in the vagina. Only a small proportion of these (less than 200) actually get anywhere near the egg. The rest either drain from the vagina or are killed by hostile conditions in the vagina, cervix or uterus. The heartiest sperm gain entry to the fallopian tube within 5 minutes of ejaculation and are helped on their journey by involuntary contractions of the uterus and the dipping motion of the cervix during female orgasm. They can survive for up to 72 hours so that intercourse does not have to be timed precisely in relation to ovulation. Once in the vicinity of an egg, the sperm undergo a process known as capacitation, which involves a series of chemical and structural changes that make them fertile and enable them to penetrate the egg's outer shell.

what are my chances?
25 per cent of unprotected sex result in pregnancy in the first month, 60 per cent within 6 months, 75 per cent within 9 months, 80 per cent within a year, 90 per cent within 24 months.

go for it!
Many couples who are trying to conceive make the mistake of waiting to have sex until they feel the woman has already ovulated. This may be too late. It is better that the sperm be on their way to intercept the egg prior to ovulation, so that the single fertilising sperm is already there when the egg is on its downward journey through the fallopian tube. The sperm have time on their side and can wait. Their normal life span is 48–72 hours, whereas an egg lasts only about 24 hours.

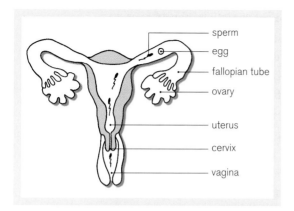

sperm
egg
fallopian tube
ovary
uterus
cervix
vagina

BEFORE FERTILISATION

For fertilisation to occur successfully, there must be an adequate number of normal sperm in the right place at the right time, there must be no obstructions in the uterus or fallopian tubes and ovulation of a normal egg must also have taken place.

Following ovulation, the egg sticks to the surface of the ovary, surrounded by a layer of cells that attract the open end of the fallopian tube. The fallopian tube's finger-like projections sweep across the surface and collect the egg from it. Once in the tube, the egg is wafted towards the uterus by other fine finger-like projections (cilia), which beat in the direction of the uterus.

For fertilisation to occur, this process must go smoothly and a number of other conditions must also be met. Not only must the number and quality of the sperm be adequate, there must also be clear passage for the sperm up through the cervix and uterus and for the egg from the ovary through the fallopian tube. There can be no physical obstructions. Ovulation must also occur at the anticipated time, and conditions in the egg must be favourable. Once fertilisation has occurred, the blastocyst (the earliest stage in the development of the embryo following fertilisation) must implant in the wall of the uterus and grow so that the pregnancy continues and does not end in early miscarriage—a surprisingly common event.

Age and fertility

Age has a profound effect on fertility, particularly for women. Natural fertility declines after the age of 25, slowly at first and then more rapidly after 35. By the age of 40, approximately 40 per cent of women are infertile, while after the age of 45, the chances of conception are less than 10 per cent. Male fertility also declines with age although not to the same extent. This discrepancy may be because the testes continually manufacture new sperm, whereas the ovaries contain their full quota of eggs at birth and when the menstrual cycle starts, usually around the age of 11, one egg is discharged each month.

main causes of infertility

Him

low sperm count and motility
retrograde ejaculation
blockage of vas deferens

Her

ovulating irregularly or not at all
fibroids
endometriosis
large ovarian cysts
blocked fallopian tubes

Diet and fertility

One of the biggest single dietary deficiencies linked to fertility problems in both men and women appears to be zinc. Zinc affects almost everything to do with reproduction, particularly the longevity of the sperm. It also plays a vital role in cell division and hormone balancing. One sign of deficiency is white marks on the fingernails.

Women who drink seven or more cups of coffee a day are almost twice as likely to have problems conceiving. Tea, on the other hand, can improve the chances of conception. Californian scientists claim the benefits of xanthenes in tea (which improve the egg's health) far outweigh the negative effect of the caffeine in the drink.

Investigating and treating infertility: men

If you and your partner are having trouble conceiving, you should consult your doctor. He or she will recommend a series of investigations in an effort to pinpoint the problem.

As far as the male half of the equation is concerned, a semen analysis is the primary investigation. For this, your partner will be requested to produce a sample of semen into a specimen jar, which is then brought to a laboratory for analysis. The analysis has to be completed within a few hours of production or else the sperm may die. Also, the sample should be carried in contact with the body to maintain warmth. Usually the sample is produced by masturbation, in the clinic where the analysis is carried out.

The semen analysis looks at the number and quality of the sperm in terms of how they move and what proportion are normally formed.

Semen samples can vary considerably from week to week so if the first test results show irregularities another sample may be requested. If this is also abnormal, the patient will be referred to a urologist for further assessment. The urologist will examine the testicles looking for a varicocoele, or varicose vein, which can raise the local temperature and so decrease sperm production. Other anatomical features will also be assessed, for example the doctor will check that there is no blockage of the vas deferens (the tube that connects the testicles to the seminal vesicles). Another potential problem (found in 1 out of every 100 men) is retrograde ejaculation at the time of orgasm, which sends semen back towards the bladder rather than along the urethra. Blood tests may also be done to see if your partner produces antibodies that destroy his own sperm and to measure his hormone levels. Past injuries and infections will also be discussed as they could be of particular relevance.

How to improve sperm

A number of causes, including environmental ones (pollution and diet), have been blamed for the dramatic decline in the Western world's sperm count and motility (the way the sperm moves) this century. Sperm health can be improved by a few simple measures:

- Stopping smoking and drinking caffeine in excess
- Cutting back on alcohol consumption
- Wearing loose underwear and trousers
- Some research suggests selenium and zinc supplements may help with motility and count respectively.

smoking and sperm

'Men with a low vitamin C intake have a markedly increased likelihood of genetic damage to their sperm. Cigarette smoke is high in oxidants and depletes the body of vitamin C and other antioxidants. Levels of a marker indicating genetic damage to sperm cells were found to be 50 per cent higher in smokers than non-smokers.'
The Nutritional Health Bible by Linda Lazarides

Investigating and treating infertility: women

For women, the initial investigation consists of a history and physical examination. The doctor will ask you how old you were when your periods started, whether you have painful periods or bleeding between periods and will discuss other relevant issues such as pain during intercourse. Questions may also be asked about weight gain or loss (extreme weight loss or gain can affect estrogen levels and ovulation), headaches, problems with eyesight, discharge from the breasts, medications, previous surgery (particularly to the abdomen or pelvis) and any previous pregnancies. The physical exam will consist of a general assessment but will focus on the presence of normal secondary sex characteristics such as breast and genital development. An internal pelvic examination will determine the position of the uterus, detect any tenderness and locate possible ovarian cysts and fibroids. A cervical (Pap) smear may also be performed.

Ovulation

Initial blood tests will normally include a measurement of your prolactin and progesterone levels in the second half of your menstrual cycle (during the 14 or so days after ovulation). Prolactin is the hormone that stimulates milk production. An excessive amount of it outside pregnancy may cause breast discharge and inhibit ovulation. If there is also a swelling in the gland that produces prolactin, you may have headaches and disturbances of vision. Some studies suggest stress may increase prolactin levels. Progesterone is measured in the second half of the cycle following ovulation because it normally increases after ovulation has occurred and a rise in levels is indirect evidence that ovulation has occurred in that cycle. Conversely, a low level suggests ovulation is not taking place.

Other blood tests include your FSH (Follicle Stimulating Hormone) and LH (Luteinising Hormone) levels. These two hormones are involved in the process of ovulation and are useful in determining your ovaries' possible receptivity to stimulation. Their comparative levels are also useful in diagnosing polycystic ovary syndrome (PCO). PCO is a condition associated with irregular periods, excessive hair growth and often excess weight gain. The ovaries are full of tiny little cysts that represent the arrested development of eggs. When infertility is the problem PCO is usually amenable to treatment with drugs to stimulate ovulation, Clomid being the usual one prescribed.

Ultrasound may also be used to assess whether or not you are ovulating. The scan is performed mid-cycle, around the time just preceding ovulation, to see if a follicle, a small fluid-filled cyst on the surface of the ovary from which the egg is extruded, has formed. Another scan is performed a few days later to confirm that the follicle has disappeared. If it has and the serum progesterone level is elevated, you have ovulated.

Your ovarian reserve test, AMH (anti-Mullerian hormone), will also be performed. This gives an indication of how well your ovaries will respond to treatment should you need IVF. The test also indicates whether or not time is on your side.

Fertility drugs

Your doctor will prescribe fertility tablets if there is evidence you are either not ovulating at all or not ovulating regularly. Clomiphene is the 'basic' fertility drug and is often effective taken at its lowest dosage. The normal starting dose is 50 mg per day for five days, starting between days 3 and 5 of the cycle (day 1 being the first day of bleeding). There is a slightly increased chance of conceiving non-identical twins when taking the drug—two eggs may be produced and both may be fertilised. Apart from this, side effects are rare.

More powerful drugs to induce ovulation are available but must only be taken under strict medical supervision because of the possibility of over-stimulating the ovaries and causing multiple cysts to form. This hyper-stimulation syndrome, although uncommon, may make a woman extremely ill, but is rarely fatal.

The pelvis and ovaries

The next step is to assess the pelvis internally, sometimes by laparoscopy. This procedure is performed under general anesthesia during which a fine telescopic camera is inserted through the navel allowing a comprehensive view of the pelvic area (uterus, ovaries, fallopian tubes) to be seen on a television monitor. The operating gynaecologist will be looking particularly for signs of endometriosis, adhesions, evidence of infection and/or blockages of the fallopian tubes.

The gynaecologist will use laparoscopy to examine the ovaries. Ideally, the procedure should take place mid-cycle or early in the second half of your cycle so that signs of ovulation may be observed. A sample of the internal lining of the uterus, an endometrial biopsy, may also be obtained at the time of laparoscopy by performing a d&c (dilatation of the cervix and curettage). In this procedure, the neck of the cervix is stretched and a sample of the lining of the uterus is scraped away and sent for analysis. The fallopian tubes are checked by passing sterile water tinged with blue dye through the cervix into the uterus and out into the tubes. If no fluid passes through the tubes, an x-ray of the uterus and tubes, a hysterosalpingogram, may be taken at a later date. This will pinpoint where the blockage is and help in planning further therapy. Sometimes, for no apparent reason, fluid may not pass through the tubes at laparoscopy but the x-ray is normal and confirms

Karen's story

Karen (36) is a secondary school teacher, as is her husband. After one try they decided IVF wasn't for them.

'I found all the various procedures terribly disturbing. It was all so invasive and there were so many different stages at which things could go wrong. After it was over and unsuccessful I felt guilty that I didn't want to go through it again. The counselling was very helpful and convinced me that I was doing the right thing by not trying again; they helped me to see that it was a positive thing to have tried at all and that no one should expect me to try again, including myself. Once I really did believe I'd given it my best shot I was able to move on to ultimately accepting that we wouldn't get pregnant and now we are trying to adopt instead. In my heart, I know we've made the right decision.'

that the tubes are in fact open. The same procedure, using ultrasound instead of x-ray may be suggested as an alternative. A hysterosalpingogram is often the first step nowadays, instead of a laparoscopy.

Fibroids

Benign muscle tumours, or fibroids, are extremely common, affecting 20 per cent of women over 30. Most do not cause any problems but if they are large or in a bad place, they can have an effect on fertility. They may inhibit implantation or prevent the blastocyst from reaching the uterus by compressing the fallopian tube. If they are thought to be causing problems, they can be removed surgically, leaving the ovaries and uterus intact.

Endometriosis

Endometriosis is a condition associated with painful periods, sometimes deep pelvic pain during intercourse and infertility, though the exact relationship between the disease and infertility is not always clear. In endometriosis there are areas in the pelvis, sometimes appearing as spots, which behave like the internal lining of the uterus and bleed at the same time as menstruation occurs. This bleeding and the associated inflammatory response of the pelvic tissues is thought to be the cause of the pain. Endometriosis may cause extensive adhesions in the pelvis and may block the fallopian tubes. It may also interfere with the ovaries and in some cases may interfere with fertility in an as yet unknown way. Not every woman with painful periods has endometriosis, indeed most don't—just as not every woman with endometriosis, no matter how extensive, is infertile.

If you have endometriosis, it may be treated either surgically or medically, depending on the circumstances. Medical treatment consists of giving anti-oestrogen drugs that cause an artificial, temporary, menopause-like state. This hopefully will cause the endometriosis to shrivel because it is not stimulated by oestrogen. Treatment usually lasts for 3–6 months, after which another laparascopy may be required to assess the condition of your pelvis.

Cysts and adhesions

Surgery may also be required if you have large ovarian cysts or if your fallopian tubes are blocked for any other reason—perhaps by pelvic adhesions. The success rate will depend on the extent of the adhesions and/or the nature of the blockage.

relieving the stress of infertility

In her book, *Healing Mind, Healthy Woman* (Dell) Dr Alice Domar relates her experiences as the founder of a counselling group for infertile women in Boston. She has developed a stress management/therapy program to help women confront life after being diagnosed as infertile—to help them rediscover sex just for fun, diaries without ticks for when ovulation is expected, happiness without positive test results. Not only did patients flourish under her guidance, she was surprised to find that within six months of completing the program, 44 per cent had conceived. Women with the highest levels of psychological distress about their infertility were far less likely to conceive than those who weren't as depressed. Although she started out just trying to improve her patients' quality of life, Domar demonstrates that relieving stress in the lives of severely depressed infertile women may also increase their chances of becoming pregnant.

IVF

If these treatments fail, or if irreversible blockage of the fallopian tubes is the cause of infertility, you may wish to try in vitro fertilisation (IVF), or test tube pregnancy. In IVF, fertilisation occurs outside the body, in a lab, and resulting embryos are then placed in the uterus. This is an extremely demanding process—physically, emotionally and in most cases, financially. IVF is not covered by the public health service or health insurance companies and costs several thousand euro per attempt. About 40–60 per cent of IVF couples will be successful and bring home a baby.

The IVF process involves stimulation of the ovaries, collection of eggs using ultrasound guidance, fertilisation of the eggs in the laboratory and the placing of the fertilised eggs in the uterus. The best results are achieved if no more than two embryos are replaced; ideally only one embryo is replaced. Embryos are assessed using an embryoscope which detects the most healthy embryo for placement in the uterus. What to do with the remaining embryos is a complicated legal and moral issue. There is no simple answer. It is standard current practice in many places to freeze surplus embryos so they are available for future transfer, allowing the couple to forego the first part of the gruelling IVF process the next time round.

If you are considering IVF you will attend informational lectures and counselling before starting treatment. Both you and your partner should be sure that you are ready for the treatment before you commit to it. Try to develop realistic long-term goals in the context of your life together.

it may work both ways

Liz and Mike came back from working in New York to start a restaurant in Galway at the same time as they were trying to start a family.

'My husband and I stopped using contraception after we got married and although we weren't trying to have a baby we were having sex and still not getting pregnant. I joked about how much money I'd wasted on the pill over the years. After a while, though, it occurred to me there might be a problem but we didn't see anyone about it until two years had gone by since I had stopped the pill.

Investigations didn't turn up any conclusive reason for our infertility, which was both maddening and reassuring at the same time.

We did our first round of IVF in America and were unsuccessful. When we moved back to Ireland, the somewhat less salubrious surroundings of the Dublin clinic took some getting used to (especially for my husband). I was very distracted by the move and wasn't expecting to get pregnant after the first go, which was probably a good thing in retrospect. The whole procedure was definitely easier the second time when even if the surroundings were different the procedures were somewhat familiar. I got pregnant just as we were setting up our business so I was good and distracted. Normally I would have obsessed about the pregnancy but I just didn't have time. When our IVF baby was 18 months old I got pregnant again naturally and irony of ironies, had to go back on the pill. Now when I look back on that period in our life, it feels like it all happened to someone else—I think maybe I consciously detached myself from the realities of what was going on then so I could get through it.'

IVF timeline

1 A full investigation into the cause of infertility is conducted before IVF is considered. An ultrasound scan is performed to assess the accessibility of the ovaries for egg collection.

2 The clinic arranges counselling prior to treatment to confirm your suitability for the programme.

3 The ovaries are suppressed at the beginning of the treatment cycle, which begins within days of the period. Large doses of hormones are administered, either by sniffing an aerosol preparation every four hours, or by regular injection.

4 Approximately two weeks after suppression commences, an ultrasound scan and blood test are performed to confirm suppression has been successful. If the ovaries have not been suppressed, medication continues for a further week.

If successful, egg production is stimulated by another series of injections while the original suppression medications continue to be taken. The aim is to enable the lab to harvest more than one egg.

5 On the night before egg collection, an injection of another hormone, Human Chorionic Gonadotrophin (HCG) is given to mature the eggs.

6 Egg collection is achieved by passing a fine needle into the follicles, which are located by ultrasound. This procedure is done on an outpatient basis. The father then supplies a sample of semen, which is treated in the lab to provide optimal conditions for fertilisation.

7 The collected eggs are placed in a special nutrient for up to 24 hours and then mixed with the sperm. Both are then incubated. If fertilisation occurs, it is visible within 18 hours.

8 Approximately 48 hours after egg collection, the embryo(s) are transferred to the uterus.

9 Embryo transfer is done by threading a fine tube into the uterus and injecting the embryos through it. Further hormone injections may be prescribed over the following two weeks.

10 Two weeks following the transfer, a pregnancy test will confirm whether or not the embryos have implanted successfully. Another two weeks on, it may be possible to visualise the developing embryos with ultrasound. If implantation has not been successful, vaginal bleeding will probably begin soon after.

Other techniques may be appropriate in some cases.

Sperm donation

Sperm donation means artificial insemination by donor and is practised by some clinics. If you are contemplating this technique you will need skilled counselling before commencing treatment. Donors are screened for a variety of infectious diseases such as HIV (AIDS) and hepatitis. An effort is made to match physical characteristics as closely as possible to your partner, but clearly this is not always possible. In a small society such as Ireland, semen may be imported to minimise the risk of inadvertent insemination by a relative.

Egg donation

Egg donation involves another woman donating an egg from her ovaries, which is then fertilised as in IVF with your partner's semen. The resulting embryo is inserted into your womb to develop as a normal pregnancy. The process involves both you and the donor undergoing the IVF procedures outlined above on an almost 50/50 basis. The donor will need to be stimulated to produce the eggs and you will need to have your uterus artificially prepared to receive and nurture the developing embryo until the placenta takes over the process naturally.

Egg donation also requires extensive counselling before it is undertaken. You must be comfortable with the fact that you will be carrying someone else's genetic material as well as with the procedural demands of the treatment.

IUI (Intrauterine Insemination)

In this treatment, sperm are injected directly into the uterus using a fine tube attached to a syringe. Egg production may need to be stimulated in a similar way to IVF although the drugs prescribed rarely need to be as powerful. This is a fairly straightforward procedure but is less likely to be successful if the female partner is over 35. Success rate: 25–30 per cent.

GIFT (Gamete Intra Fallopian Transfer)

In this process, eggs and sperm are introduced directly into the fallopian tube through a fine tube threaded through the cervix and uterus. This process is similar to IVF except that fertilisation takes place in the fallopian tube, not the lab. GIFT removes the ethical dilemma of what to do with surplus embryos. Success rate: similar to IVF. It is not commonly used.

ICSI (Intra Cytoplasmic Sperm Injection)

A single sperm is injected through the shell of the egg in the lab after the egg is harvested as in IVF. The technique is suitable for couples where the motility of sperm is poor. The success rate is higher than that of IVF and varies from one clinic to another. Compare notes if you are considering this approach.

ZIFT (Zygote Intra Fallopian Transfer)

ZIFT is similar to IVF, too, except that the zygote, or embryo, is transferred into the fallopian tube rather than the uterus, and at an earlier stage. This technique attempts to mimic normal pregnancy by placing the early embryo in the fallopian tube where fertilisation usually takes place. It is very rarely used nowadays.

Marion's story

Marion (32), a solicitor and her husband have been trying to have a baby for three years while also juggling demanding careers.

'At the outset my partner and I agreed that we would give IVF three chances. We felt it was important to put a limit on how long our lives could be on hold. My husband is a doctor and knew full well, too, how emotionally and physically demanding IVF is and that there was only so much we could go through. It was particularly hard for me to put work on hold whenever I needed to and to give issues at work my full attention when I was swimming in hormones and feeling awful. Finally, I had to explain to my colleagues what was going on so they wouldn't wonder why meetings were being cancelled and I was suddenly taking days off when there was a lot on. They were very understanding throughout.'

Carmel (34) is from a large family and has eight nephews and nieces. She coped with the ups and downs of two rounds of IVF (the second successful) by keeping busy—going to the gym before work, taking classes at night.

'When you're in an IVF program, the hormones make you feel awful—it's like having the worst PMT imaginable, all the time. You feel sad, angry and acutely sensitive to anything people say, particularly about babies. And it's inevitable at my age that talk turns to kids all the time. Friends and relatives who know what you're going through try to be sensitive but sometimes their efforts get to you. You try to stay positive and put things into context but sometimes you just can't. One thing that really got to me was that after the first attempt failed, everyone immediately started talking to us about adoption. They were trying to be helpful but it hurt. I found that during the treatment it was better for me to keep time chatting with them over coffee or drinks to a minimum. We'd go see a funny movie or something instead. A little escapism really helped.'

After fertility treatment

Many women who get pregnant after fertility treatment are very apprehensive about losing the pregnancy and even when everything goes well, the pregnancy may seem unbearably long and demanding. The emotional challenges and strains of fertility treatment require incredible stamina and inner strength, even when everything goes according to plan.

Try to remember that once you are pregnant your risk of miscarriage is only very marginally greater than in an unassisted pregnancy. Take it as easy as possible. Allow yourself as much breathing space as possible in terms of extra commitments because you will be under considerable mental pressure, particularly during the first three months of pregnancy. Even if you try hard not to be preoccupied with your pregnancy, it will never be far from the forefront of your mind and you will need time and support to refocus your goals. Only then can you be comfortable with your new situation and begin to enjoy your pregnancy.

If treatment is not successful, you should evaluate whether or not you should try again with the help of a qualified counsellor. Having done it once, you will be better able to make an informed decision about whether or not you would like to undergo another round of IVF. Try to remain objective as best you can about what is right for you and your partner and your life together. This has to be a joint decision.

Frequently asked questions

Does smoking affect fertility?
Heavy smoking (more than 20 cigarettes a day) can inhibit both the quantity and quality of sperm. A decrease in sperm motility is the main effect of heavy smoking. As far as women are concerned, research from the University of California at Berkeley has found that a woman who smokes 1–9 cigarettes a day may decrease her fertility by as much as half.

I have not been using birth control for two years and although I have been having sex regularly, I'm beginning to wonder if there's a problem. Should I consult a doctor?
Yes, if you are concerned at any stage after six months, talk to your doctor.

Is there an age limit for IVF programmes?
No, but many programmes concentrate on couples in which the woman is under 40. This is because the treatment's success decreases with advancing maternal age.

Are IVF pregnancies more risky?
Only slightly, because of a higher chance of multiple birth. An IVF pregnancy is, however, less likely to be allowed to go overdue.

I have been placed on a large number of drugs following successful IVF. Are they all really necessary?
Evidence to support the taking of anything other than progesterone supplements in early IVF pregnancy is scanty to say the least. Most clinics do not recommend steroids (prednisolone) or anticoagulants (heparin or aspirin) or indeed anything other than progesterone.

How successful is IVF?
Overall success rates in terms of bringing home a baby, are around 50 per cent. Beware of statistics claiming higher success rates as they may be including 'chemical pregnancies' where you have a positive pregnancy test but subsequently miscarry. Success rates are higher in younger women, under 35 years (60+ per cent), and lower after the age of 40 (40+ per cent).

11 when things go wrong

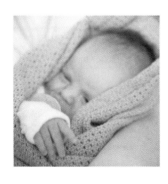

Although the vast majority of diagnosed pregnancies result in a healthy baby, sadly, even with all the benefits of high standards of care and modern medicine, things still go wrong. Some babies die before or soon after birth; others are born with life-threatening disease or serious but not potentially fatal conditions.

Where mothers are concerned, Ireland is one of the safest places in the world to give birth. Although deaths do occur, usually from conditions unassociated with pregnancy such as brain haemorrhage (which might have happened even if the woman had not been pregnant) or cancer, sometimes the death can be caused by specific complications of pregnancy such as haemorrhage, or a clot in the lung. Occasionally, for a variety of reasons, a pregnancy or labour may cause physical or emotional problems for a mother after the birth. Most conditions either resolve themselves with time or can be successfully treated.

Risks to the baby

The main risks to the baby in pregnancy are of miscarriage in the very early stages of pregnancy, and death later in the pregnancy. A normally formed baby, that is with no major abnormality such as spina bifida, who has reached 24 weeks of pregnancy, has a greater than 99 per cent chance of survival. This should be a great source of comfort and reassurance. The chances of congenital malformation of a major life-threatening type are approximately 2 per cent. Examples include failure of the kidneys to develop, severe heart malformations or hydrocephalus. Other less grave malformations such as club foot or cleft palate occur in another 2 per cent so that the total risk of malformation is approximately 4 per cent.

Babies may also be born with various chromosomal disorders, of which the most common is Down syndrome. Some neurological abnormalities such as cerebral palsy may only become apparent some months after birth.

The risk of a baby dying before birth, for no apparent cause, is approximately 1 per 1000. This is similar to the risk of sudden infant death or cot death, for which there is also no known cause.

Even with the great advances in neo-natal care, babies who are born very prematurely, 14 or more weeks before term, have little chance of survival.

will my baby be healthy?

Once you have gone beyond 24 weeks and your baby does not have a major abnormality, you have a 99 per cent chance of having a healthy baby. If your baby is born with a serious condition medical staff will help you to chart the best course of action for your child's care and help you to cope with the enormous additional challenges confronting you and your partner.

Miscarriage

The most common thing to go wrong with pregnancy is miscarriage. If you have a miscarriage you will understandably be very upset. There are some things that are important to understand as you try to cope with your grief. First, there is absolutely nothing you could have done either to prevent the miscarriage or cause it. Unfortunately, going to bed or not working are no help; the outcome has been determined at conception. If you are leading a reasonable lifestyle, miscarriage is beyond your control. Smoking very heavily or taking drugs—especially cocaine, which causes spasm of the blood vessels—can increase the chances of miscarriage, but nothing else in the course of normal daily life can. Stress does not cause miscarriage.

Almost every woman who has a miscarriage focuses on something she feels she should have done or not done as being responsible for the miscarriage. This guilt is entirely misplaced. Advice from others to rest at home when a miscarriage threatens is well intentioned, but of no medical benefit.

Most miscarriages occur early, before 12 weeks. These early miscarriages are usually due to problems arising at the time of conception when the sperm and egg join together. At this stage there is great potential for things to go wrong and if they do, the result is that the embryo dies—in other words a miscarriage takes place. This process is completely beyond anyone's control, especially yours. At the time of conception the survival chances of a baby are virtually pre-ordained.

How the genetic code works

At conception there is a complex exchange of genetic material. The genes which make up chromosomes 'instruct' each cell in the body how to function, develop and combine with other cells to form the various body organs such as bones, heart, brain, etc. Even a small alteration in the way genes are laid out can cause significant problems. The genetic code can be regarded as a recipe for the human body—an extraordinarily complicated recipe—but a recipe nevertheless! As an example of the way a small alteration can cause problems consider the following recipe:

'Take two eggs and mix with one tablespoon of flour.'

If this recipe, or genetic code, is altered by the deletion of one letter, say the 'k' in the first word 'take', and all the words remain the same length the code will read as follows:

'Taet woe ggsa ndm ixw itho net ablespoono ff lour.'

A relatively simple instruction becomes virtually meaningless. So even a small change in the genetic code can result in serious problems in development and function. Down syndrome babies, for example, have just one extra chromosome (number 21) and the resultant problems are clear for all to see.

Indications of miscarriage

The first sign of a miscarriage is usually bleeding, which will prompt you to attend hospital and your carers will organise an ultrasound scan. From 6 weeks after the first day of your last period, it should be possible to see a foetal heartbeat on scan. If the embryo is seen but the foetal heartbeat is not, it may mean that your pregnancy is not far enough advanced to detect one. In that case another scan may be scheduled for the following week. If a foetal heartbeat is seen, then your bleeding will be classified as a threatened miscarriage.

More often, the signs of a miscarriage are first apparent between 8 and 10 weeks after your last period and a scan will show a dead embryo, which may be smaller than expected. If the embryo is only 7 weeks' size, for example, but you are 10 weeks into your pregnancy it does not mean that your baby died at 7 weeks. What it means is that your baby had some very serious condition, which proved fatal, and impeded growth by at least 3 weeks.

Sometimes a scan will reveal an empty sac and no embryo. This may be because after death the embryo effectively dissolves back into the fluid-filled sac. In the very early stages of development there is no bone formation and the consistency of the embryo is similar to jelly. After death the tissues lose their firm consistency and melt away. For the same reason it is not unusual for no embryo to be seen after the miscarriage is completed, whether with or without d&c.

If the embryo has died and you have not passed any tissue, you have had a missed abortion or miscarriage. If some tissue has been passed, it is an incomplete miscarriage. If everything has come away, it is a complete miscarriage.

If the embryo has died and you have not passed all of its tissue, the doctor will probably advise you to have a d&c, usually under general anaesthetic. Typically, this involves a day in hospital and will be arranged as quickly as possible. Any bleeding should settle within 2–3 days of the procedure.

If miscarriage occurs very early in pregnancy, say at 7 weeks, you will be given the option of going home to complete the miscarriage on your own. The advantage of this is that you are spared a general anaesthetic and a day in hospital; the disadvantage is that you may find it more emotionally distressing and you may ultimately require a d&c anyway if your uterus fails to expel everything. You should discuss your concerns and options thoroughly with your doctor.

possible signs of miscarriage

Most miscarriages occur before week 12. After this, the risk of miscarriage is very low. Call your doctor or go to hospital if you experience any of the following:

- bleeding with cramps or abdominal pain (pain on one side at less than 9 weeks could be a sign of ectopic pregnancy), especially if you have a history of miscarriage
- bleeding as heavy as that of a period or light staining that lasts three days or more
- severe abdominal pain that lasts more than one day even if there is no bleeding.

An ultrasound scan will clarify matters for you. If there is a heartbeat and the embryo is a normal size at 6 weeks from your last menstrual period you have a less than 1 per cent chance of miscarriage.

When a d&c is performed, all tissue is usually sent to a lab for analysis. Despite this, it is rare to find a specific cause for miscarriage, even if chromosomes are successfully grown and analysed from tissue samples. Chromosome analysis may sometimes reveal the sex of the embryo. It is not standard practice to attempt to grow chromosomes from tissue obtained at the time of miscarriage, partly because it is rarely successful and partly because the facilities to do so in a large number of cases are not available in this country. The other reason for analysing tissue is to exclude a hydatidiform mole (see A–Z chapter).

If the foetus dies later in pregnancy, but before 24 weeks, your baby will probably be delivered vaginally because a d&c is not appropriate and may be dangerous. In these circumstances, it is normal practice to induce labour using a form of prostaglandin pessary or by taking tablets. Labour is usually much quicker than at full term and delivery is physically less demanding. Unfortunately, the placenta is often retained so you may require a d&c afterwards.

miscarriage and stillbirth

Miscarriage is the death of an embryo, foetus, or baby, very early in the life span, before 24 weeks gestation.

The vast majority of miscarriages occur before 12 weeks.

Stillbirth occurs when a baby, of at least 24 weeks gestation, dies before birth and is then born dead.

Stillbirth

Stillbirth is when a baby of at least 24 weeks' gestation dies before birth and is then born dead. There are a huge number of reasons why this can happen but in practice it is rare, occurring in less than 1 per cent of pregnancies. Sometimes, a baby will die for no apparent cause, similar to sudden infant death. This can be very frustrating and frightening because there is no explanation for the death. In other cases, death may be due to malnutrition because the placenta does not function properly. This problem is frequently detected during antenatal visits before the baby is in danger because the baby is smaller than expected.

If your baby dies before birth, your immediate reaction may be to ask for a caesarean. This is not recommended because it entails a major operation that will leave you with a scar on both your skin and the uterus. The latter could have implications for future pregnancies and the whole physical recovery process could slow your emotional recovery. You will have enough to cope with without further physical discomfort following delivery.

It is likely that your labour will be induced if your baby dies before birth, although some women prefer to wait for labour to begin spontaneously. Prostaglandins are used in these situations although the particular prostaglandin used is more powerful than that used closer to term. While the physical aspects of giving birth are the same as if the baby were alive, there are naturally dramatic emotional differences between the two experiences. Hospital staff will try to anticipate your needs as best they can and be sensitive to them. The baby will be given to you to hold after delivery and you should take plenty of time together—the hospital will allow you as much time together as you want, both immediately following the birth and in the days to follow. Most people keep the baby with them for 24 hours and then make funeral arrangements but there is no norm to comply with. Do whatever you feel is best. The midwife will photograph the baby for you but you may also take pictures if you wish.

After delivery, you will be taken to a private room in the hospital, which will hopefully be out of the earshot of crying babies, although sadly this is not always possible in a busy maternity hospital. You will usually stay in for a couple of days but if you want to go home earlier, hospital staff will do their best to facilitate this. It may be no harm to stay in hospital even if your instinct is to return home to familiar surroundings and family. If you have other children at home, it may be difficult to get as much rest as you need to begin coping with the trauma of losing your baby. Generally, it is not recommended to rush funeral arrangements. They can wait until you are feeling stronger.

When you are ready, it is worthwhile that the baby has a full autopsy. You will be able to see the baby again afterwards and the baby will not look damaged. Sometimes, the autopsy can help clarify why the baby died, which could be important for future pregnancies. Some laboratory results will be available quickly, but others, involving more complex tests, may take several weeks. The placenta or afterbirth should also be examined as it may provide an answer as to why the baby died.

Neo-natal death

Neo-natal death is defined as death within 28 days of birth. Most neo-natal deaths are due to severe prematurity—babies who are 10 weeks or more premature have a much higher mortality rate. A very premature baby has some chance of survival from 24 weeks onwards. There have been huge advances in neo-natal intensive care in the past decade and these advances are continuing apace. Perhaps a decade from now, the lower limit of viability will have been extended even further.

Because modern intensive care facilities are so good, it may take several weeks for a baby to die. This is a very traumatic experience for parents. They must watch their baby struggle, attached to life support systems, and they must endure the full gamut of emotions as the baby's condition often seems to improve for days only to collapse unexpectedly.

coping with a baby's death

One of the hardest aspects of a baby's death, whether you have suffered a miscarriage, stillbirth or neo-natal death, is dealing with people's comments about the will of God, fate etc. When you first get your period again, you may be very upset because it is a reminder that you are no longer pregnant but have no baby. The time when the baby should have been born if you have had a miscarriage, or anniversaries of stillbirth, birth and death, may be especially trying. Don't fight your feelings, but do bear in mind that once your period has come again your body is ready to try again.

Counselling and support are available in most parts of the country and specialised groups like the Miscarriage Association of Ireland and Irish Stillbirth and Neonatal Death Society (ISANDS) are open to everyone, including extended family. Many hospitals provide counselling, too, particularly for later deaths. It can be enormously helpful to talk things through with both professionals and other people who have been through similar bereavements.

Don't forget that although your husband/partner has not suffered a physical trauma he has also suffered the emotional trauma associated with a baby's death.

Among more mature babies who die in the neo-natal period, the more common reasons for death include lack of oxygen at birth due to abruptio placentae, where the placenta breaks away, or prolapse of the umbilical cord. Both are quite uncommon conditions.

Some rare chromosomal abnormalities are almost invariably fatal, usually in the first week of life. The two most common of these are trisomy 18 (Edward's syndrome) and trisomy 13 (Patau's syndrome). Babies born with Edward's are very much smaller than average and have some subtle differences in appearance, which are sometimes only noticed by experienced paediatricians. If there is a suspected problem, a blood test will be ordered and sent for analysis. Babies with Edward's rarely survive more than a week and are often stillborn. Babies with Patau's are also smaller than expected and have 'rocker bottom' feet with convex rather than concave arches and other superficial abnormalities. Far more serious are their internal abnormalities, which are usually too debilitating to surmount.

Still other babies die because of congenital malformations or for completely unexpected reasons—infection or Sudden Infant Death Syndrome (cot death).

Infection in an otherwise healthy infant is unusual and may be due to meningitis or pneumonia acquired in the womb or during the course of delivery. Infection with listeria is also a possible cause of death although it usually causes death to occur before delivery. In a full-term baby, infection as a cause of death is extremely rare—infection does occur but it is usually treated successfully.

if your baby gets sick

Babies who get sick in the first six weeks of life are still technically outpatients of the maternity hospital in which they were born and will be treated by the doctors there. If there is something wrong with your newborn, every effort will be made to ensure that you understand exactly what your baby's condition is at all times.

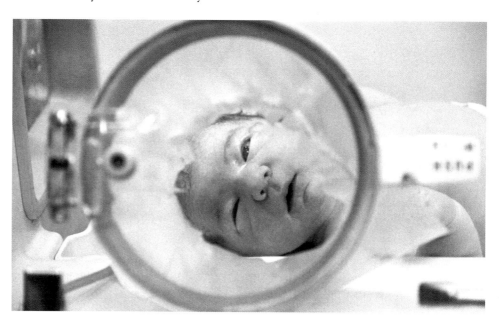

In the following sections I give a brief overview of some of the more serious conditions seen in newborns.

Cerebral palsy

Cerebral palsy is a neurological disorder, usually diagnosed within the first year of life. It is characterised by stiffness of the muscles and abnormal movement. There is a huge range of disability associated with CP. Some people are only mildly afflicted, with stiffness in just one leg, while others find every muscle in the body including the neck, head, arms and legs are affected. In 50 per cent of cases, CP is accompanied by some degree of intellectual disability. In other words, half of those who suffer from cerebral palsy have normal intellectual abilities.

The incidence of cerebral palsy in the Western world is 2 per 1,000 births. This may be higher than you would expect but the figure has remained largely unchanged for the past 30 years. On the positive side, if your baby is born at full term, the odds against cerebral palsy are 500 to 1.

There is no real way of knowing before birth if your baby is going to develop into a normal, healthy baby but the odds are certainly favourable.

In most cases, the causes of cerebral palsy are unclear but probably date back to conception. A small number are due to difficulties during childbirth. It is difficult to say exactly how many are due to this cause because often babies who have a pre-existing problem (which it is not possible to know about) will only behave abnormally for the first time during labour or in the newborn period.

Less than 10 per cent of cases are identified as having been caused by complications of birth and many of these are associated with extreme prematurity where the baby is born before 28 weeks. Sometimes these births are complicated by haemorrhage from a separating placenta or infection from membranes that have ruptured very prematurely. In general, however, the risk of premature birth in Ireland is very low, less than 5 per cent, and most of these premature births are closer to 36 weeks than 28 weeks so that death and disability from complications of birth are quite rare.

In most cases, mental and neurological problems will only become apparent with the passage of time. If a baby has no difficulties in the immediate newborn period (the first week of life), long-term difficulties are extremely unlikely. Even if babies show signs of abnormal behaviour, like seizures, they are still more likely to develop normally than to have an intellectual disability.

Half of the babies born with cerebral palsy have normal intelligence; the other half have intellectual disability of varying degrees. As your baby grows, it may become extremely difficult to manage his or her care on your own, both physically and emotionally. In Ireland, if your child is diagnosed with CP you will be referred to Enable

Ireland (01 261 5900 www.enableireland.ie), where you will meet with professional carers—doctors, nurses, counsellors, physiotherapists and teachers—as well as other parents and children whose lives have been touched by CP. Together, you can plan for the future.

Chromosomal problems

There is a myriad of possible genetic problems that can arise out of the blue at the time of conception. If you have a family history of genetic abnormalities, draw this to the attention of your doctor before you try to get pregnant or early in the pregnancy. Many chromosomal problems are random events however, and will not be detected until the baby is born.

Having a baby with a chromosomal problem is never easy. You are bound to have very mixed feelings. Couples' reactions vary from complete rejection of the baby to complete acceptance and it is not unusual to go through the whole range of feelings in the immediate aftermath of delivery. It is incredibly difficult to grieve for the loss of the normal baby you had anticipated having, while at the same time bonding with your new baby and trying to understand what special demands his or her care will place on you.

what exactly is Down syndrome?

A normal baby has 46 chromosomes and a pair of sex chromosomes (XX for a girl, XY for a boy). The most common chromosomal abnormality is trisomy 21, or Down syndrome, which occurs once in every 700 births and is due to the baby having an extra chromosome 21. The superficial characteristics of Down syndrome are a flat nose, partially closed eyelids (particularly close to the nose), loose skin at the back of the neck, and a single crease across the palm (as opposed to three—look at your own hand). The baby's muscle tone is also usually reduced so that they appear more 'floppy'. More importantly, the baby will suffer from some degree of intellectual disability. The extent of it will only become apparent as the baby gets older. It can vary considerably from child to child.

Down syndrome is usually apparent immediately after birth but with some babies it is difficult to diagnose until it can be confirmed by a blood test, which can take up to 3 weeks. The only definitive way to diagnose it antenatally is by amniocentesis or chorion villus sampling, which can be performed between 11 and 13 weeks.

There are two types of Down syndrome. The most common is non-inherited, a random occurrence. The second, rarer form is known as non disjunction of chromosome 21 and this may be inherited through the mother. If there is a strong family history of Down syndrome in your family, you may want to test to see if you are a carrier before conceiving.

A small percentage of babies with Down syndrome are stillborn. Just as a baby with Down's has a much higher likelihood of being stillborn and may die unexpectedly at the end of pregnancy, so babies with Down syndrome also have a higher incidence of congenital abnormalities, especially of the heart. Having said that, babies with milder forms of Down syndrome in which their heart is not affected have no greater risk of dying in the newborn period than babies without Down syndrome.

Guilt at feeling disappointed by your baby's condition is a normal response and may be exacerbated by the dramatic hormonal changes you will be undergoing after the birth. You may also find that your feelings are out of synch with your partner's and may find this very distressing.

Most communities and hospitals have excellent support systems and offer counselling for parents confronted with the responsibility of caring for a child with Down syndrome and other chromosomal disorders. Listen to their advice and let them help you both short and long term.

Physical abnormalities

If your baby is born with a physical abnormality you and your partner will feel understandably shocked and concerned. Sometimes the abnormality is immediately obvious, as in the case of spina bifida or cleft lip. In other cases, the abnormality may not become apparent for days or even weeks after birth. Some congenital heart conditions show no abnormal signs until the baby develops heart failure at a few weeks of age. Other heart abnormalities, like a hole in the heart, may be diagnosed by the paediatrician during the baby's first physical examination after delivery.

Neural tube defects

In normal circumstances, the spinal cord closes in the first 4 weeks following conception. If any part of the cord fails to close, spina bifida results. The most severe form involves the baby's skull and brain directly, and is known as anencephaly. The most common form involves the lower back, where the spinal cord may be exposed or may only be covered by a thin fluid-filled membrane like cling film. The mildest form is effectively hidden and may only be represented by a dimple in the middle of the lower back. This mildest form has no effect whatsoever on your child's development, whereas the most severe form, anencephaly, is fatal.

Spina bifida is an uncommon condition that is made less likely by taking folic acid supplements before you get pregnant and in the first few weeks of pregnancy. Both it and its most serious variant, anencephaly, can be diagnosed by ultrasound after 16 weeks, sometimes before. Therefore you are likely to be aware of a problem, if one exists, before the baby is born. You will be told if your baby has a neural tube defect at the time of the scan. If you would like a termination of pregnancy you will be advised to travel, probably to a unit in the UK. Termination of pregnancy is not legal in Ireland unless the mother's life is in danger. If you decide to continue with the pregnancy, you will be supported throughout it by your medical team and a paediatrician will be involved with the baby's care very soon after birth.

The extent of the baby's problems will become more apparent after birth, when your baby will be attended by both paediatricians and neurosurgeons in order to determine the best course of action. Surgery may be required in some cases. If the spina bifida lesion is severe you may be advised to have terminal care for the baby rather than attempt surgery, which could make the baby suffer unnecessarily.

Congenital heart disease

Congenital heart disease can be very difficult to diagnose before birth and frequently is not recognised until after a baby is born. A hole in the heart is usually not as severe a problem as it sounds and often will cause no problems whatsoever. Almost every baby looks blueish or purple immediately after birth but usually within a few minutes its colour becomes pink. Don't worry if your baby's colour isn't perfect immediately.

If the paediatrician suspects a problem, further tests will be ordered under the supervision of a consultant paediatric cardiologist, which may involve the transfer of the baby to a paediatric hospital. If the baby needs surgery it may be deferred until the baby is bigger and better able to cope with surgery. Technically, it is easier for surgeons to operate on a bigger baby because at birth a baby's heart is only the size of a plum.

Kidney problems

Abnormal development of the kidneys can range from complete failure to develop to minor anatomical differences such as obstruction to the flow of urine from the kidney to the bladder. The less severe problems will often settle in time, as your baby grows. Other more severe problems may occur as a result of blockage of drainage of urine in the womb and in some cases foetal surgery may be advised to temporarily relieve the blockage before the baby is born. Sometimes a suspected problem with the kidneys will noted on ultrasound but, by the time the baby is born, the problem may have resolved itself without intervention .

Cleft or hare lip and palate

While it may be a tremendous shock to you when you first see your baby, it is important to remember that cleft palate and hare lip, which usually go together, are completely curable with cosmetic surgery. The results of these operations are superb: following surgery in the first year of life even babies born with severe cleft palate and hare lip will look completely normal. Failure of the palate to develop properly often runs in families and is sometimes diagnosed antenatally, but it can be very difficult to visualise the baby's mouth area with ultrasound. If it is diagnosed, you will be told.

Babies with severe cleft palate may require tube feeding initially. Breastfeeding will be impossible, although you may arrange to express milk for the baby's bottle feeding.

Possible problems for mothers

Problems affecting you as a mother, rather than your baby, can arise at any stage of pregnancy, and those problems can be either physical or psychological. In this section I deal with problems that may arise during labour and after delivery. For example, you may be disappointed that your labour and the birth haven't gone as expected. You may have ended with a forceps delivery or caesarean section when what you were expecting was a smooth, normal delivery. The key to coping with your disappointment is to have realistic expectations about the birth and to keep an open mind as labour unfolds.

Every birth is different. If you are concerned in any way about your experience ask for an explanation. Doctors and midwives are on your side and keen that you have a good understanding of what happened. If you don't ask the questions they may be unaware that you are unhappy, so do ask. If your expectations are not fulfilled it may predispose you to the development of postnatal depression, so do make sure that you discuss any problems you may have and be aware of the possibility of depression.

Complications of caesarean section

In Ireland your chances of having a caesarean section on your first baby are 20 per cent or more, but this figure varies significantly from one hospital to the next. If you are concerned about this possibility you should try to check it out before you book for delivery, although of course this is not always a realistic proposition if you live in an area where your choices are limited. The reasons for caesarean in labour are usually either concern about your baby's condition (foetal distress), or because your labour has come to a halt and there is no further progress (dystocia or failure to progress). Before labour one of the commonest reasons is because the baby is coming bottom first (breech).

Apart from a sense of failure if you were hoping for a normal birth there are a couple of things that can go wrong, either during the section or after. The worst that could happen is that during the section there is so much bleeding that you have to have a hysterectomy. Thankfully this is very rare and in practical terms is not something you should consider a cause for real concern. On a first birth in particular this is even more rare. If you have had a caesarean on your first birth, however, it is slightly more frequent and the risk increases with each successive caesarean delivery. This is primarily because the placenta may implant itself under the scar from a previous caesarean and be impossible to remove in the normal way after the baby is born.

Because a caesarean section is a surgical procedure (operation) inevitably more blood is lost during the birth. While this is usually not a problem it may leave you especially tired after the birth at a time when you need all your energies to look after your new baby, and of course yourself. If you know in advance that you are going to have a section make sure your iron levels are well in the normal range. The best way to do this is to take supplemental iron during your pregnancy. If you lose a significant amount of blood during your surgery you may be so anaemic afterwards that a blood transfusion may be indicated, and while this is an extremely safe procedure it is something to be avoided if at all possible.

A caesarean delivery leaves you with a scar on your abdomen and, quite apart from the extra pain, you are at risk of developing an infection in the wound. An infection will cause swelling, redness, and painful inflammation around the wound. This can delay your recovery and will require antibiotic treatment. Thankfully this is not a common experience.

A scar on your uterus has implications for your future births. While it is safe to try for a vaginal delivery on your next if you have had only one caesarean the chances of success are reduced to approximately 80 per cent, as opposed to greater than 95 per cent if your first delivery was vaginal. There are also long term implications gynaecologically in that a scar on your uterus can cause difficulties if you ever need to have a hysterectomy – not something you are thinking about at this stage I hope!

Episiotomy problems

With a vaginal delivery there are also a series of possible problems. If you have an episiotomy, or a tear, that requires stitches the area can become infected, the stitches can break down or 'unravel', or the area can heal abnormally with residual pain severe enough to make intercourse impossible and require a small operation to cure it.

Your chances of requiring stitches on a first birth are approximately 50 per cent, whether you have an episiotomy or not. The fewer the episiotomies that are performed in a hospital the higher the rate of perineal tears. Almost all stitches inserted nowadays are dissolving and so don't need to be removed.

An infection will show itself by pain, redness and swelling more than the norm. If in doubt ask a midwife, or the district nurse, to have a look at it. Don't put salt in the bath to improve healing; it won't help but it will make it more painful. Antibiotics will be prescribed if there is clearly an infection. It is unusual for the stitches to unravel so that the episiotomy breaks down. If it does happen you will probably need to have it redone, possibly under general anaesthetic, or maybe a spinal anaesthetic so that you can be awake.

The pain from an episiotomy should get progressively less in the days and weeks following delivery. At six weeks you should have virtually no pain or even discomfort. The area is very well equipped to heal well. A normal part of the healing process in the first few days after delivery is for the area to swell, and this can be quite painful but should resolve by the third day. If you are still having a lot of pain at six weeks mention it to your doctor; it may be that an abnormal healing process has gone on, either with too much scar tissue or the edges haven't aligned themselves correctly. In any event you may need a small procedure to 'redo' the episiotomy and this is usually completely successful.

Urinary problems

Sometimes it may be impossible to pass water after delivery. This problem, urinary retention, is not common but can be quite distressing. It is more common after an instrumental vaginal delivery, after a caesarean section, or if you have needed catheterisation during labour, for example with an epidural. Urinary retention is by no means inevitable after any of these but is certainly more frequent than if you had an uncomplicated delivery without an epidural.

As a general rule the longer the labour the more complicated it becomes and the more likely you are to have difficulty passing water. If you do develop retention you will need to have a catheter placed, probably for at least 24 hours, after which bladder function will usually return to normal.

Urinary incontinence occurs when you leak urine if you cough or sneeze, or rarely if your bladder gets so full, without your being aware of it, that it overflows. The risk of long-term problems with bladder control is around 30 per cent, lower with a caesarean section. The risk is increased with long labours, pre-existing bladder control problems, or if you are overweight. Pelvic floor exercises are helpful in reducing your risk of urinary incontinence long term.

Damage to the anal sphincter (back passage)

Damage to the anal sphincter, which controls defecation (passing a motion), can cause the distressing symptom of inability to control the back passage, causing involuntary passage of faeces or flatus. While this can be a problem immediately after birth the good news is that the majority of cases resolve over the weeks and months following delivery. Sometimes physiotherapy may be necessary, while in rare cases surgery may be necessary. If you are still having symptoms six months after delivery it is unlikely that they are going to resolve without intervention.

The damage occurs either during the delivery by tearing of the muscles, or by nerve injury from compression by the baby's head in the birth canal in the time leading up to delivery. The risk of symptoms developing is less than 10 per cent on a first birth, and less than 5 per cent on later births. The risk with a caesarean section performed during labour is less, and less again with a caesarean performed before labour. Risk factors for the development of damage include forceps delivery, a long labour, and a large baby.

If you have any of the symptoms of damage do make sure to tell your doctor, don't be embarrassed. The symptoms are distressing but can be cured.

Anal tear

There is an uncommon condition, fissure in ano, which sometimes occurs in association with childbirth, particularly if there is constipation also. The symptoms are severe pain when passing a motion, often with some bleeding also. It can usually be treated successfully with suppositories which your GP can prescribe for you. Rarely it may require a small operation.

Retained placenta

The placenta normally separates within minutes of your baby being born. It peels off the inside wall of the uterus like a large postage stamp on the inside of a collapsing balloon. The placenta is made up of many individual units and normally they all come away together. Occasionally the whole placenta stays attached and may have to be removed by hand by the doctor. If you have an epidural in place it can usually be done with the epidural providing sufficient pain relief; if not you will probably need a short general anaesthetic. Sometimes one of the small units may stick to the inside wall of the uterus and be retained. If this happens it usually declares itself by excessive bleeding in the days after delivery although sometimes there may be few signs for a week or so, and then there is more bleeding than expected. If this happens you will almost inevitably need a general anaesthetic to remove the adherent fragment.

Post partum haemorrhage

Excessive bleeding after your baby is born is called post partum haemorrhage. Normally the bleeding should get progressively lighter in volume, and darker in colour, and then stop completely. Your uterus will normally contract tightly, like a muscle in spasm, and this has the effect of closing off the blood vessels in your uterus and stopping the bleeding. Within days of delivery the bleeding should be getting darker and by two or three weeks will probably have stopped completely.

If you breastfeed you may find that you get episodes of fresh red bleeding from time to time, and these can occur up to eight weeks after delivery. You only need to be concerned if the bleeding is persistent and heavy, enough to soak a maternity pad every 20 or 30 minutes. Clots are the result of blood collecting inside the uterus, forming a clot, and then being passed out of the uterus. The passage of clots is often accompanied by a gush of fresh red blood. Clots of themselves don't mean that the bleeding is excessive.

Excessive bleeding that occurs immediately after delivery may be due to failure of the uterus to contract correctly. The injection given after birth to help the placenta separate is also helpful in preventing this type of post partum haemorrhage. It may also be due to retention of the placenta, which will be obvious to your caregivers. Occasionally it is due to trauma to the birth canal, almost always associated with an operative delivery--forceps or vacuum.

Haemorrhage occurring more than 24 hours after delivery is usually due to either infection or a retained piece of placenta. Infection is associated, sometimes but not always, with a fever, foul smelling vaginal discharge and an abnormally tender uterus which is not shrinking back to normal size at the appropriate rate. Treatment is with antibiotics which may need to be given intravenously and therefore require a stay in hospital for a day or two. Breastfeeding can continue, even if you need antibiotics. If the haemorrhage is due to a piece of placenta which has stuck to the inside of the uterus you will require an anaesthetic to have it removed and you should be fit for home the next day.

If you are at all concerned about the amount of bleeding you should contact your doctor or the hospital. It can sometimes be confusing as to whether the amount is normal or excessive. If in doubt, ask!

Symphysiotomy

Sometimes the tendons joining your pubic bones loosen causing a slight separation of the pubic symphysis joint. When the two bones rub together this can cause great pain. The ligaments may even sever completely, causing a spontaneous symphysiotomy (see page 56). The condition virtually always resolves itself with time as the tendons heal without intervention. Physiotherapy can be a great help in facilitating your recovery.

Mastitis

If you breastfeed you may contract an infection called mastitis which can be caused by germs getting into a cracked nipple. This should be treated as quickly as possible to prevent it developing into an abcess. You can develop mastitis without a cracked nipple, however, and not every woman with a cracked nipple gets mastitis. If you suffer from a fever, localised redness, swelling, flu-like aches, nausea and vomiting, see a doctor immediately. Once treated with antibiotics, the infection usually begins to subside in 24 hours. You should feed through the illness even if it is painful. Doing so will not harm your baby but it will help you. The infection is in your breast, not your milk and not feeding will only lead to engorgement and possibly blocked milk ducts or abcess formation.

Postnatal depression

Having a baby is a massive life event. Your first child turns you from being a daughter to being a mother, overnight. It is a daunting prospect to look after a vulnerable, new little human being in whom you have invested so many hopes and dreams. It is no wonder that the emotional stress can sometimes precipitate a feeling of helplessness, inability to cope and frank depression. The most important aspect of postnatal depression is to recognise that it might be affecting you. The worst thing you can do is to deny the possibility that it might be affecting you.

Postnatal depression is no respecter of age, class, intelligence, level of education, achievement in career before pregnancy, or type of birth. Everyone is susceptible. Having said that, it is not very common and you, as an individual, are unlikely to get depressed. A degree of 'baby blues' is not uncommon, especially in the first couple of days after the birth. There is an inevitable feeling of anticlimax for some mothers after the birth but this should pass within days.

Signs of depression to watch for include crying for no apparent reason, not wishing to see anyone other than your baby, sometimes not even wishing to see your baby, extreme tiredness along with an inability to sleep, lack of interest in your appearance, and a feeling of not being able to cope with your baby. If you feel that you may be either depressed, or developing depression, make sure you get help. There is nothing to be ashamed of and you are acting in an extremely responsible way, both to yourself and to your baby and partner, if you acknowledge that depression may be developing. The good news is that it is very treatable, sometimes with counselling and sometimes with medication for a period of time. If you had a pain in your tummy that interfered with your life you would surely want it fixed; think of depression as a pain in your spirit, and remember–it's fixable.

Frequently asked questions

My friend's baby was born very prematurely and died 6 weeks ago. She has still not seen any of her friends or a counsellor and I worry that she may not be coping. Is there anything I could be doing for her? Will a counsellor contact her if her family doesn't contact them?
You should encourage your friend to contact her GP, who will be able to assess the situation and make the appropriate referral if needed. The hospital where the baby died will have made an appointment for review in any case, but normally a counsellor would not contact her.

I am having a scan tomorrow because my baby seems small for the dates. If the baby is small what will happen? Will I be induced straight away? Will the baby be at higher risk for things going wrong?
What happens will depend on a whole variety of factors, including your stage of pregnancy, whether or not the baby is in fact small or just seemed that way on examination in the clinic, and how small the baby is. The ultrasonographer and/or doctor will discuss everything with you at the time of the scan.

12 younger and older mothers

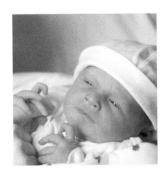

Most pregnant women in Ireland are between the ages of 30 and 37. In the National Maternity Hospital in Dublin in 2014, 71 per cent of all mothers were between the ages of 30 and 39 (that represents more than 6500 mothers). There were more than 3500 over the age of 35—the age at which mothers are medically defined as older—and 631 aged 40 or over.

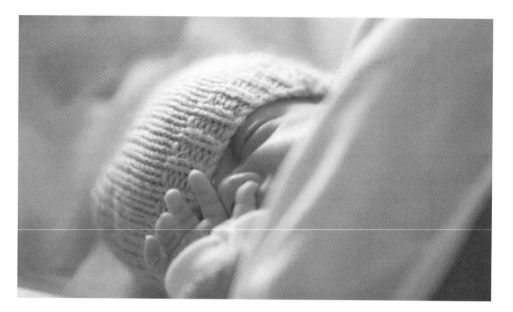

Younger mothers

Discovering that you are unexpectedly pregnant in your teens can be terrifying. You may not believe that the pregnancy test is correct and may need to take a second test to convince yourself of the result. Try not to panic and try to share the information with an older person whom you trust, preferably your parents. If you don't feel ready to talk to them, a teacher or another family member may help.

Your family doctor is likely to be very understanding and helpful and will not break any confidences you share with him or her. You may prefer to talk to another doctor who does not know you and your family. Doctors are trained to deal with your situation and will be very sympathetic and understanding. Remember there is virtually no situation that your doctor has not encountered before. Your situation is not unique, has happened a million times before and will happen a million times again in the future.

If there is no one you feel comfortable talking to, you can speak in absolute confidence to: +OPTIONS 1850 62 26 26 www.positiveoptions.ie

You are probably going to be pleasantly surprised by how understanding and supportive people will be about your pregnancy. There are not so many social stigmas about being pregnant and unmarried as there were in the past. Your parents may be extremely upset at first but their concern for your welfare should be foremost. After the initial shock they will hopefully rally to your side. If they don't, adjusting to your pregnancy will be very hard for you and you may need counselling all the more.

Once you know that you are pregnant, your future course of action depends on some big decisions. You will be greatly helped in making your decision by professional counselling available from +OPTIONS.

Your pregnancy

The good news is that physically, teens do very well in both pregnancy and in labour. From the time that you can get pregnant, your body is ready to have a baby. There are no extra complications associated with being pregnant young.

It may be hard for you to make the lifestyle changes you should make if you are still a teen. You must try to stop smoking and being in smoky places and you should avoid drink altogether. Cigarettes, drugs and alcohol are bad for your baby and it is your responsibility to take good care both of the baby and yourself. It is also your responsibility to attend your antenatal clinics and visits so that any potential problems in your pregnancy can be detected early.

Some mothers worry that their pregnant daughters will have a difficult pregnancy because their pelvises are so small but medically, this is rarely a problem. Labour and delivery are normally fine, with many younger mothers finding that an epidural helps keep them from being overly frightened by the whole experience. It is important to remember that all kinds of pain relief are available to all mothers and that you will never be left alone while you are in labour. You will be well supported by a team of midwives and can bring someone with you to keep you company during labour. If you are thinking about bringing a friend however, try and bring someone who has been through labour themselves. Professionals in the hospital will do everything they can to make the experience easy for you.

don't skip class

For every woman, pregnancy is a learning experience. Antenatal classes are designed to help you understand exactly what is happening and what will happen to your body during pregnancy and labour. You should attend all these classes because they will help you to understand what is happening to your body. The more you know, the more confident you will feel. Your friends will have horror stories about people they know who have had babies; the more you understand about pregnancy the more you'll be able to take these with a grain of salt, as most of them are grossly exaggerated.

After your baby is born the midwives will show you how to feed and bathe your baby. You should also visit a social worker in the hospital early in your pregnancy so they can explain what benefits you are entitled to.

Antenatal care

With regard to antenatal care, you should attend your hospital or doctor early so you can plan for what is going to happen during and after the pregnancy. You may need a scan to determine when you are due if you are unsure about when your last period was. It is important to know exactly when your baby is due because you may need to plan changes in your study timetable or change your exam times. Schools and colleges will try to accommodate you and will usually postpone your exams if they fall late in your pregnancy or right after your baby is born. You need to discuss these issues with your teachers or lecturers. Being pregnant doesn't mean that you have to miss out on educational opportunities. After you have had your baby you should try to return to finish your studies. Many schools and colleges now have creche facilities. If they don't you will need to make alternative plans for childcare well in advance.

Try breastfeeding

After your baby is born, you should try to breastfeed, especially while you are in hospital. Breastfeeding has a lot of advantages over bottle feeding. First, breast milk is the best food your baby can have from a health point of view. It will help your baby stay strong and healthy. Second, it's very convenient. You will always be able to feed your baby as long as you are with him or her—you can go anywhere without bringing anything with you—no bottles, sterilisers or formula. You won't have to get up in the middle of the night to make up a feed. And finally, breastfeeding costs nothing. It is easy to breastfeed without other people noticing if you are worried about being slagged. It is easy to do it quietly without anyone even knowing or seeing what's going on (although they may hear some happy gurgling noises from somewhere under your shirt). Breastfeeding does not make your breasts sag afterwards. If there is an effect on your breasts it is from the pregnancy, not from feeding the baby.

Single parenting

If you are not in a long term, stable relationship you may find that the father of your baby virtually disappears and refuses to have any involvement with you or your baby once he discovers you are pregnant. This can be terribly hurtful, but unfortunately it happens all too often. Even if your pregnancy was planned, the pregnancy may place a strain on your relationship as it brings new responsibilities with it. Try to handle situations sensitively, particularly when you are telling him you are pregnant. Pick a time and place, don't blurt it out in anger or in front of other people.

Sarah's story

Sarah was in her final year of school when she found out she was pregnant. She didn't tell her family for three months until her mother confronted her. 'I tried not to gain much weight so my parents wouldn't notice because I was afraid to tell them. When I did they were really angry. My mother said she knew they'd end up minding the baby all the time and that I was only doing it to get out of doing the Leaving. We didn't talk for a week but then when my boyfriend scarpered we made up. She went with me to the hospital when I had Jack and that was great. I had an epidural so it wasn't too sore but the stitches were agony and I hated being so fat. I didn't go out for a month after Jack was born because I looked so bad. I don't go out half as much as I used to now because my Mum won't mind the baby every night but she minds him if I'm at work and if I go back to school I'm sure she'll look after him. I miss being able to do whatever I want whenever I want.

If you don't have supportive friends and family who can help soften the blow of a break up, it is important to remember that there are many organisations who offer free counselling and advice. They exist because they want to help. You do not have to try and cope on your own before or after the baby is born.

Adoption

If you do not feel confident about raising a child yourself, you may want to consider putting your baby up for adoption. This decision will require extensive counselling, which is available through the social work department of the hospital you attend. Alternatively, you can get help through +OPTIONS.

Although not chosen as often now as in the past adoption can offer a very positive solution to your dilemma. If you find yourself pregnant and in a position where it will be virtually impossible for you to care for the child yourself adoption provides a positive alternative to termination of pregnancy. You can be sure that the couple adopting your child will provide a loving environment. Adoptive parents undergo a very detailed screening process before they are approved for adoption by the relevant agency. The process is a lot more open nowadays and there is legislation in place which will ensure that you will be able to know how your child is developing over the years if this is your wish. If you wish to establish contact with your child in the future this will be arranged if both parties, you and your child, are agreeable to this. In some circumstances you may have the opportunity to meet the adoptive couple.

While giving up your baby for adoption may be the toughest thing you ever do in your life you are giving your baby a chance of a full life and you are giving a couple the opportunity of a family that they might not otherwise have had.

Abortion

If you cannot cope with being pregnant and you and your parents have decided you are going to have an abortion, you will need to get proper professional counselling. This can be arranged through one of the agencies in +OPTIONS. The abortion will not be performed in Ireland but you will be given phone numbers of clinics in Britain or mainland Europe. It is not legal to actually make the appointment for you. Because of language problems and the familiarity of British clinics with your circumstances coming from Ireland, it is best to opt for the British route.

The procedure of abortion, or termination of pregnancy (TOP), is similar to a d&c where the opening into the womb, the cervix, is stretched or dilated (the 'd') and the womb is emptied or curetted (the 'c'). The operation is usually, though not always, done under general anaesthesia and you are discharged the same day. When you return home you should have a check-up to confirm there have been no complications—you can make arrangements for this before you leave hospital.

If you decide to have an abortion, the earlier it is done, the better. It is progressively more difficult both medically and emotionally from 12 weeks onwards although in the UK it is legal to have a termination up to 24 weeks.

Physically, an abortion presents few dangers or risks to you or your future fertility. Emotionally, an abortion can have a major effect on you and the memory of it will stay with you for the rest of your life. The physical strains it will place on you are minor but the emotional ones can be huge. For this reason it is terribly important that you get adequate counselling from someone who has been trained to deal with the emotional issues specific to abortion.

Contraception

As soon as you resume having sex after your baby is born you should be taking birth control if you don't want to get pregnant again. Discuss what kind is best for you with the midwives while you are still in hospital. They can arrange any necessary prescriptions before you go home.

Older mothers

The medical profession has traditionally defined the older mother as 35 or over, based on the fact that from 35 onwards there are some increased risks to both mother and baby that are directly related to age. However, more and more women are choosing to start their families later or are continuing to build them well into their 40s and the vast majority do so without encountering any major medical setbacks. If you are over 35, you will nonetheless have some different concerns about your pregnancy that you should feel free to air at antenatal visits and classes.

Late starters

Your natural fertility declines progressively from its peak in your early 20s and this decline accelerates after 35. You may therefore find it more difficult to get pregnant in your late 30s. The reason why your fertility declines after 35 seems to be related to the health of your eggs. From the time your periods begin, one egg is released every month and it appears that the healthier eggs are released earlier in life. In theory the oral contraceptive pill may be beneficial in 'storing' eggs in a state of suspended animation, so if you have been on the pill for years some of the natural decline in your fertility may be offset. This is pure conjecture however and there is no good scientific evidence to back it up. Fertility declines to the extent that by your early 40s it is down to approximately 10 per cent.

The risks

Once you are pregnant, you have an increased risk of miscarriage if you are over 35. This is because there is an increased risk of chromosomal abnormalities such as Down syndrome, which can result in the very early death of the embryo—in other words, a miscarriage. It is difficult to put a figure on the risk of miscarriage because each pregnancy is unique. In any case, while the risk of miscarriage increases, you are still much more likely to have a normal pregnancy than for a miscarriage to occur.

The increased risk of Down syndrome is directly related to advancing maternal age. At age 30 the chance is 1 in 850, at 35 it is 1 in 350 and at 40 it is 1 in 100. Because of these increased risks, you may wish to have tests done to see if your baby will have an abnormality.

If you opt for testing it does not mean that you are going to have a termination if the results are not what you had hoped. The purpose of testing is to give you information that will enable you to make choices about how you wish to handle your pregnancy. Termination may be an option but it is only one option. Testing may reveal a treatable condition that can be remedied before the baby is born (or soon thereafter), or it may enable you to prepare for raising a child with a disability more effectively. In the vast majority of cases, testing simply reassures parents that all is well and facilitates a more relaxed pregnancy.

An early scan for nuchal translucency, combined with a blood test, that evaluates your individual risk of having a baby with a chromosomal abnormality is widely available here. You may well have to have a non invasive pre-natal test, NIPT (see page 32). There is no risk whatsoever associated with having a scan. After you receive your test results and your doctor explains them, you may also wish to have amniocentesis or chorion villus sampling to determine conclusively whether or not your baby is affected.

Do keep in mind however that amniocentesis and chorion villus sampling carry a risk of miscarriage that wouldn't arise if you didn't have the test. You need to have thought through clearly why you want the test and what you would do if the test result is not normal.

Age does not increase your risk of having a baby with a congenital abnormality, other than those due to chromosome problems. Spina bifida and congenital heart disease are not more common with older mothers.

crisis pregnancies—older mothers

If your unexpected pregnancy represents a crisis for you, you should seek advice about what your options are by contacting one of the agencies listed under +OPTIONS. They are skilled in helping pregnant women through crises, not matter what you ultimately decide to do.

General health

From your point of view, if you are physically strong and healthy and are not suffering from any long-term conditions like high blood pressure or diabetes, pregnancy itself will not present any major increase in risk to your own health. You will have a slightly increased chance of developing diabetes during pregnancy (gestational diabetes), or high blood pressure confined to the pregnancy (toxemia), but in general, these risks are low.

As you get older, you will probably be less tolerant of the discomfort and even aches and pains that are part and parcel of a normal pregnancy. Accept this and make lifestyle changes in anticipation of the limitations pregnancy will place on you. In other words, take it easy. You can plan on continuing your normal activities as much as possible—keep up exercise (swimming is especially beneficial), keep working, but don't be surprised if you feel tired and need extra rest. That doesn't have to be a negative; many women enjoy relaxing into their pregnancies.

Labour

If you have delivered vaginally before, labour and delivery should present no major challenge to you just because you are over 35. If it is your first baby, labour is usually tough no matter what your age (and will make you stiff and sore for a few days). You may have an increased chance of induction and caesarean, primarily because your doctor will probably be unwilling to take the slightest risk and will probably intervene more quickly than if you had given birth to a healthy baby already without any problems. In other words, if you have a good track record, things may be handled slightly differently. These are issues you can discuss with your doctor or midwife.

The fitter you are going into it, the easier labour is likely to be. In general, if you are older you will be likely to ask better questions and be better able to put things into context. You're also likely to know and understand your body a bit better than younger mothers, and you will probably be a bit more assertive about your care, too. Doctors are often happier dealing with people who know what they want!

After the birth

Physically, you should not have any more difficulty with any aspects of being a new mother than someone younger. Emotionally, there may be some advantages to being more mature. You'll probably be better able to figure out your own limitations and, hopefully, won't try to take on too much immediately after the baby is born. And if you've already had children before, you'll know that infancy passes all too fast and you'll try to make the most of your time together with the new baby.

Frequently asked questions

My boyfriend is too scared to come to the birth with me and I don't want my mum there. Can my friend come?
Yes. You can decide who you want to be with you. You can even have a relay of a few people with you if you wish—but only one at a time. Choose someone mature who has preferably given birth themselves. If you want to be on your own, that's fine too—a midwife will be with you at all times anyway.

I'm about halfway there and I haven't been to the clinic yet. My friend says they don't do anything but weigh you and take some blood anyway. Does it matter if I don't go for a while?
Yes, it does matter. There may be some problem you may not be aware of. Do you know you're not having twins? Are you anaemic? Go early and stick with the programme—it is designed for you and your baby's benefit.

I am 39 and pregnant with my fourth baby after a gap of five years. I feel very different this time—exhausted and emotionally drained. I've had amniocentesis so I know the baby is physically well but I'm tired just thinking about what's ahead of us and I worry about the gap between the baby and the others. What can I do?
Physical exhaustion is easily dealt with—listen to your body and rest whenever you can if you feel you're overdoing it. Emotional exhaustion is more complex. There is no doubt that finding out that you are pregnant unexpectedly can be a major shock. You are probably settled into a routine and enjoy 'having your mornings back' when the older children are in school. Giving that time up represents a big sacrifice. Meanwhile, keeping everything at home ticking over takes a lot of energy and you wonder how you'll find enough extra to juggle a baby as well. These are understandable reactions but try not to dwell on them without taking action.

Use the months ahead to make adjustments in your home life that will make things with a baby more manageable. Gradually get the older children and your partner to take on a few more responsibilities around the house, make standing arrangements for play dates and school runs so you can carve out more time for yourself and the new baby. Order your shopping on the internet, cut back on extra-curricular activities for a time. You should also consider letting your standards slip a bit for a while—everything doesn't have to be the same after the baby as it was before in terms of meals on the table and tidiness. The world will not end if you are late dropping the children into school, buy more convenience foods or don't help with the homework every day. It sounds trite but a lot of people get very wound up about relatively minor things. If you feel genuinely overwhelmed, however, talk to your GP or doctor, who can refer you to a counsellor.

After I have this baby I am sure that I don't want to get pregnant again. Should I get my tubes tied or should my husband have a snip—which is most reliable and easiest?
Sterilisation is undoubtedly the most permanent form of contraception around.

The advantage of female sterilisation is that you are 'safe' from the time of your next period. Disadvantages include the need to have a general anaesthetic to have your tubes tied. The advantage of male sterilisation (vasectomy) is that a general anaesthetic is not necessary. The disadvantage is that you may have to wait several months before the all clear is given following production of a sperm-free sample. In both cases, female and male, there are no other effects—if sterilisation was performed on a man or woman without their knowledge they wouldn't know it. The Mirena coil is a very popular choice because it offers a form of contraception almost as effective as sterilisation, is reversible by simply removing it and has the added benefit of usually making your periods lighter or stopping them altogether. It can be placed by any doctor who has had the appropriate training. If you do go with a Mirena coil, don't be frightened by the size of the box it comes in, the coil itself is very small.

I am 40 and 18 weeks pregnant with my first baby after trying for years to get pregnant. I've had the nuchal test and my risk was low but I can't stop worrying that I'll lose the baby. My doctor says so far everything is fine. Do many older women miscarry after the first trimester?
No, after the first 12 weeks your chance of miscarriage is less than 1 per cent. If you have an early scan, at 7 weeks, for example, and this shows a normally developing embryo your chance of miscarriage is less than 1 per cent.

What is the absolute earliest I can have amniocentesis?
Most doctors don't advise it before 12 weeks at the very earliest and most would be unwilling to attempt it so early because of the increased rate of miscarriage and technical difficulty. Fourteen weeks is preferred. The nuchal scan has effectively replaced amniocentesis as the first line of assessing the risk of Down syndrome.

13 fathers

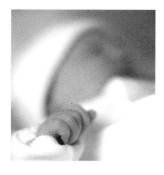

I have written this chapter for fathers. Its purpose is to provide an understanding of what pregnancy is all about without having to read the rest of the book. If you, a father, wish to delve deeper into any aspect of pregnancy you will be able to find a fuller discussion in the relevant chapter. The A to Z is likely to be of most use to you.

A life-changing event

Your wife/partner will change dramatically during the pregnancy and will not be the same person after the pregnancy, and neither will you. Your partner's changes will be both physical and psychological, your's will be psychological.

For many women, but not all, bearing a child is the fulfilment of their sense of womanhood and represents one peak of their life's ambitions. For others pregnancy is just something to be expected in the course of a life and no deeper thought is given to it. For most, pregnancy is probably somewhere in between. In other words it is a process of life changing dimensions which has a profound physical and emotional impact, not just during the pregnancy but for the rest of your life.

When a woman becomes pregnant a whole new world opens up, a world of babies, other mothers' experiences of childbirth, names for the new baby, baby clothes, the possibility of a brother or sister for the, as yet unborn, baby, fears and anxieties about the pregnancy and giving birth. Most of these thoughts will not have entered the average man's head so don't feel that you are missing some natural emotion if you are bewildered by the direction of thought of your partner. It's the beginning of a strange journey for you, the father.

Signs of pregnancy

The first sign a woman notices that she might be pregnant is when her period doesn't arrive on time. Normally they come every 28 days or so. Confirmation that she is pregnant is by a urine pregnancy test bought in the chemist's shop. Most women repeat the test a couple of times to convince themselves that it is correct. The tests nowadays are extremely reliable and accurate so if it's positive there is no doubt! The test can even be taken a couple of days before the period is due by those who are anticipating a positive result or who are anxious to find out as soon as possible. Some women know they are pregnant before they miss a period because their bodies are so finely tuned in to subtle changes, but they are very much the minority. The reaction to a positive test will naturally range from unconfined joy through to absolute horror. Either way, a positive test is undeniable.

Duration of pregnancy

Pregnancy itself is divided into three parts called trimesters. The first is from the beginning to 12 weeks, the second is from 12 to 28 weeks, and the third is from 28 weeks to the end (40 weeks on average). Confusingly, a pregnancy is dated from the first day of the last period, and not from the time of conception. So, if a pregnancy is described as 12 weeks, it is 10 weeks since conception. The normal duration of pregnancy is 40 weeks, from the first day of the last period. It is not uncommon, particularly on a first baby, for a pregnancy to last a week or more beyond the expected date of delivery, so you should be prepared for this possibility at the end.

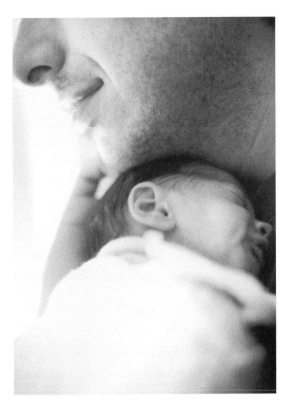

The first trimester

As soon as the fertilised egg, your future baby, has burrowed into the wall of the uterus (womb) your partner may start to notice the effect of hormone changes. The following changes may occur: her breasts will probably swell and become quite sensitive, or even sore, to touch; she may develop nausea, which isn't always in the morning; she may start to vomit up what she has eaten, or even if she has eaten nothing; constipation is not unusual and sometimes lasts the whole way through pregnancy; constipation can facilitate the development of piles (haemorrhoids), a form of varicose vein seen more frequently in late pregnancy; tiredness is often a feature of the first 12 weeks, to the extent that your partner may want to do nothing but sleep at the weekends and in the evening; sometimes the tiredness, described by some as being like bad jet-lag, can last up to 20 weeks; it is not unusual to feel some crampy pains in the lower tummy or pelvis, but they are rarely sinister; the cramps are merely the uterus reacting to stretching and growing with the new baby. The cramps are more common on a first pregnancy. Some women get headaches in the first trimester, probably due to a combination of the effect of hormones which cause blood vessels to stretch, and the fact that a woman's blood volume increases by up to 40 per cent during this period.

Almost all the changes your partner is experiencing are due to the effect of the developing pregnancy, baby and placenta, on her body, and are completely outside her control. One of the features about pregnancy that can be hard to understand, and sometimes hard to accept, is that once a woman conceives there is very little she can do to influence how the pregnancy will affect her, and indeed how she can affect the developing baby. This should be largely reassuring. For example, many couples worry that their lifestyle around the time of conception and in the very early weeks might have an adverse effect on the baby. A lot of women have been drinking alcohol and smoking in early pregnancy but it doesn't seem to cause problems for the baby. With alcohol, for example, it appears the mother has to drink heavily for prolonged periods during the pregnancy to cause noticeable problems. Even so you should remember that every time the mother has a drink so too does the baby. Most women lose their taste for alcohol early in pregnancy and this is probably a protective mechanism. The same advice holds true for smoking.

Don't be worried if your partner is unable to keep any food down, it won't harm the baby, it won't starve. A baby gets its food in elemental form as carbohydrate, protein and fat molecules, and as minerals and vitamins. These molecules are taken from the mother's bloodstream by the placenta and transported into the baby's blood across the placenta. For example, if the mother's diet is deficient in protein her body breaks down her own protein and gives it to the baby via the placenta. They really are little scavengers!

What should you be concerned about in early pregnancy?

Only two things should concern you enough to contact the hospital or your doctor: 1) if there is any bleeding vaginally, and 2) if your partner develops a pain in the tummy or pelvis that is so severe she would consider contacting a doctor even if she wasn't pregnant. Bleeding may represent a miscarriage or may be of no concern at all. The only way to clarify what is happening is to have an ultrasound scan. If a heartbeat is seen then the chances of a miscarriage are about 1 per cent or less. The very earliest a heartbeat can be seen is 6 weeks from the first day of the last period. If the heartbeat cannot be seen, and it is less than 7 or 8 weeks since the last period, your partner may be asked to return in a week's time to have another scan, particularly if there is any doubt about the accuracy of the date of the last period. This is because the pregnancy may not be as far advanced as thought. If there is no doubt about the dates and the pregnancy is at least 8 weeks or longer, and a heartbeat cannot be seen it is almost always because the baby has died—a miscarriage. Sometimes a little bleeding can occur when the placenta is developing and burrowing into the wall of the uterus. This is harmless. The important piece of information that you need is whether or not the heartbeat is present. The only way to find that out is to have a scan.

Pain in the lower tummy or pelvis is not unusual in early pregnancy, particularly on a first. It is due to the uterus stretching and growing to accommodate the growing embryo. Severe pain on one side may rarely be caused by an ectopic pregnancy (outside the uterus), particularly if accompanied by bleeding. As described with bleeding, above, the best way to clarify matters is to have a scan.

The description above of what can happen to your partner may appear daunting but be reassured, not all women experience the full range of symptoms described. Indeed some go through pregnancy hardly affected at all and wonder what all the fuss is about; others are completely flattened. Most experience some, but not all, of the symptoms and remember–they have no effect whatsoever on your baby and they settle with the passage of time. At the start of the second trimester most women have got over their nausea, their tiredness is lifting and they are feeling more human. A lot of patience and TLC is therefore required in the early stages.

Where should the baby be born?

The first trimester is the time when you should decide where the baby is going to be born and whether there is going to be full time hospital care, a combination of your GP and the hospital (the best choice in my opinion), private, semiprivate, or public care. Your GP is your best source of advice, although you will not be short of advice on all matters concerning pregnancy once the word gets out. You should ensure that your partner books in for antenatal classes early although the classes themselves don't take place till later in the pregnancy, usually from about 30 weeks on. Most hospitals will facilitate fathers' attendance at most, if not all, classes.

The second trimester

The second trimester is the 'quiet' part of pregnancy. The likelihood of something going wrong between 12 and 28 weeks is very remote so that in practical terms you can both relax. Your partner will probably start to feel the baby move from about 20–22 weeks if it's the first, earlier on subsequent pregnancies. You probably won't be able to feel the baby move until much later, from about 26–28 weeks on. You may notice your partner sitting quietly with her hand resting on her 'bump' with a dreamy, far away, look in her eyes . . . She's feeling the baby move and probably dreaming about what it looks like. Her energy will have returned to almost normal from about 20 weeks, sometimes earlier, so that you will be able to have a more normal social life. There will probably be a scan arranged for 18–20 weeks and this is one you should make every effort to attend: if you can only make it to one visit this is the one to aim for. If there are difficulties with your work or travel arrangements most hospitals will arrange an appointment to suit you both.

> Try to imagine what it must be like to be pregnant: you begin, over a period of a week or so, to feel bloated in your tummy, you have to get up twice a night to pee, you feel nauseated every morning and some days throughout the day also; some days you can keep no food down; you are absolutely exhausted and are fit for nothing in the evening, you fall asleep watching TV at 7 o'clock in the evening; the prospect of going for a pint turns you off completely; you lose interest in sex; you are constipated; you're supposed to be delighted. Congratulations, you're pregnant!

If you wish to go away on a holiday this is the trimester to aim for. Your partner is feeling more like herself, the bump is not too uncomfortable, and the likelihood of a problem while you are away is very remote. Most airlines will allow travel up to 34 weeks. Ask your doctor before you make definite bookings. In the unlikely event that the placenta (afterbirth) is lying low in the womb you may be advised against travel. Because problems are so unlikely to develop during the second trimester there probably won't be more than one or two antenatal visits during this time.

Your baby is growing and developing in the womb. It is in a very protected environment, surrounded by a cushion of shock absorbing fluid. It is effectively in an intensive care like area with the placenta acting as an artificial kidney, a lung bypass machine, and providing intravenous nutrition through the umbilical cord. The pregnancy, from this point onwards, will be hard to hide even if you wished to and so you, and your partner in particular, will be bombarded with unsolicited advice. While the advice will be well intentioned some of will be completely wrong and some will be excellent. Separating the good from the useless can be difficult, however. It's amazing how often pregnant women are subjected to others' horror stories about childbirth, often second hand, wildly exaggerated and inaccurate! Sometimes it will seem that being pregnant makes your partner public property. Some of the more common pieces of wrong advice include the following: it's dangerous to stretch because the baby's umbilical cord might strangle the baby; you shouldn't swim, run, go to the gym, wear a seatbelt, eat peanuts, sleep on your back, work at a computer screen or have sex. Believe it or not your partner is likely to hear some, if not all, of these bits of incorrect 'advice' at some stage in her pregnancy. If there is any doubt in your mind ask your doctor or midwife for guidance. The best way of dealing with unasked for advice is to say 'that's very interesting, thank you', and move on!

on the home stretch

Twenty-four weeks is a milestone. At this stage your baby weighs approximately 500 grams and is considered capable of surviving if born any time from now on. Next time you're in a shop pick up a 500 gram bag of sugar to see how much your baby weighs. If your baby is normally formed and born at any stage from 24 weeks on it has a progressively improving chance of survival , with the odds better than 99 per cent at term.

The third trimester

The third trimester begins at 28 weeks and lasts until the baby is born. Your baby is continuing to grow and making stronger and more vigorous movements. This makes them more uncomfortable for the mother. Try to imagine a large balloon expanding in your tummy. It's there 24 hours a day and puts a strain on your back as it continues to grow. Many women find it increasingly difficult to sleep as time advances. Some find they have a return of the more unpleasant symptoms of early pregnancy. Some degree of nausea is not unusual and heartburn may become pronounced so that eating may become a bit of a chore for the last month or so. Various aches and pains in the tummy and pelvis are common, and perfectly normal.

Things to watch out for

As with early pregnancy there are a few things you need to watch out for: vaginal bleeding might be serious, although it usually isn't. If any bleeding does occur you should contact the hospital, or your doctor or midwife, no matter what the hour. If it is lighter than a period (your partner will know) it is unlikely to be serious; if heavier or continuous it may signify some degree of separation of the placenta which might require early delivery of your baby. This is not usually the case, so don't panic.

Pains in the tummy or pelvis are not at all unusual towards the end of pregnancy and are rarely sinister. The pains of labour are strong enough to stop a woman walking, talking, eating or sleeping. If she can do any of these during a pain she is unlikely to be in labour. If the pains are strong enough to prevent any of these activities then she may, or may not, be in labour. The only person who can confirm this is the midwife. So, go to hospital or call your midwife.

Some women get episodes of a severe, knife-like pain, in the vagina towards the end of pregnancy. This is due to the stretching of the pubic symphysis, a joint at the front of the pelvis, which is under the influence of a hormone called 'relaxin'. The joint is composed of a band of tendon not unlike the Achilles tendon at the back of your ankle. Childbirth is a dynamic process which involves the uterus contracting, the pelvis stretching, and the baby being squeezed through the birth canal. Sometimes the pubic symphysyis overstretches, and may even tear, a condition called symphysis pubis dysfunction, or SPD for short. It is very painful, can occur before birth as well as during it, but resolves spontaneously in virtually all cases after birth has taken place.

Labour and delivery

When you go into hospital with your partner for the birth you can usually stay with her at all times if that is your wish. Nobody expects you to know anything or to take responsibility for anything so don't be scared. You will be free to ask questions and everything will be explained to you both as it happens. From the time of going into hospital until the birth occurs is usually anything from 4 to 12 hours on a first birth, but much quicker for subsequent births. You will be kept informed about progress by the midwife after each examination to see how the cervix (neck of the womb) is opening up. The pushing part of labour usually lasts about 30 to 40 minutes, but can go on for an hour or more and is hard work. Usually, if delivery is not imminent after an hour of pushing the doctor will

from purple to pink
Most babies look purple or blue when they are born so don't be alarmed by the appearance. As they take their first breaths they become lovely and pink, usually within a few minutes.

recommend some form of assistance with either a vacuum or forceps. All will be explained as it goes along and if you have attended the antenatal classes it will be much easier for you to follow what is happening. On a first birth the chances of needing help with the delivery are approximately 20 per cent but vary from hospital to hospital. The chances of a caesarean are also about 20 per cent and also vary from hospital to hospital.

Labour and childbirth are extremely stressful events but the reward is huge. Just before your baby is born you may find that your partner gets very anxious indeed and goes 'into herself'. Some women can be quite dismissive of their men at this stage and it can seem that nothing you say, or do, is right! Don't worry if this is your experience. As soon as the baby arrives all changes with the sense of relief of getting the baby out and actually seeing her, or him, for the first time. Your job is one of support and encouragement, you cannot take the pain away.

After the birth

After the afterbirth (placenta) is delivered and stitches put in, if necessary, you will be offered a cup of tea or coffee. You may not notice the placenta delivering or the stitches being inserted, because you will be preoccupied with your new 'little one', who is gazing into your eyes with a quizzical look and possibly blowing little bubbles with each breath. Enjoy it. You partner and baby will then be transported to the postnatal ward for the recovery period. On a first baby it is usual to stay in hospital for 2 or 3 days until feeding is established and your partner is confident managing your new baby on her own. If your partner is unsure about breastfeeding you should encourage her to try it and persist with it if she does start. Breastfeeding has many advantages over bottle feeding. Quite apart from the well documented health advantages there are practical advantages also—no getting up at 4 am to get a fresh feed from the kitchen, no bottles to sterilise, no bottles to bring with you when you go out, and of course it costs less.

You will find that the first weeks after the birth are a very demanding time for you both. Your partner is very tired after the pregnancy, labour and delivery. Take some time off work and help with the shopping, cooking etc. Babies are quite demanding in the first few weeks; they feed frequently, six or seven times a day or more. A feed can take up to an hour regardless of whether it is breast or bottle so there is little time for other chores. Babies soon settle into a nice routine. After three weeks you will both wonder how you ever lived without your baby. The whole experience is wonderful and greatly enhances you both as people. It can also bring you very close together.

Congratulations: you are now a father.

14 caring for your new baby

Dr John F. A. Murphy
Consultant Neonatologist, Department of Neonatology, The National Maternity Hospital

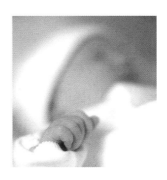

The long-awaited moment is here and the birth is over. Your newborn baby is wet, light purple in colour and partially covered in a cheese-like substance (vernix) that looks like a foundation cream. You hope he or she is normal and you wonder if you can see any family resemblances. Remember, this baby is a completely unique individual. Although he or she has bits of you, bits of his or her father and to a lesser extent other family members, the combination adds up to someone very different. It is this uniqueness that makes rearing a child so fascinating.

Getting breathing started

If your baby is slow to breathe a little bit of extra help is needed. (This is called a low Apgar.) In this event your baby will be taken to the nearby resuscitation trolley and given suction and oxygen to establish breathing. There is no need to worry about lack of oxygen—the bag and mask take over the breathing functions and your baby continues to get adequate oxygen. As soon as breathing is well established he or she will be handed to you. If a more complete check-over is needed your baby will be brought to the special care baby unit.

the special care baby unit

About 10 per cent of newborn babies need to spend time in this unit. Many newborns have minor conditions that respond rapidly to a few days' treatment. Others are born prematurely and require a longer stay. Any baby born before 37 weeks is considered premature. Sick babies and those who are very premature require neonatal intensive care.

The newborn baby examination

Your newborn baby will be given a routine examination by a paediatrician on the first or second day after birth, depending on the hospital's routine. The purpose is to establish that your baby is both externally and internally healthy and normal. The external points include skin, facial structure, eyes, limbs and hips. The internal points are the heart, lungs, abdomen and brain. Detecting problems early gives the best chance of effective treatment.

A variety of common, non life-threatening disorders can be identified on physical examination including hip dislocation, talipes (club feet), extra digits, cleft palate, undescended testes, heart murmur. If your baby has any of these conditions specialist treatment will be given as appropriate. All of these conditions respond well to treatment. At the examination a number of measurements are recorded such as your baby's length and head circumference. The head is measured because it gives an estimate of the size of the brain. The average length of a newborn baby is 51 cm (20 inches) long and the average head circumference is 35 cm (14 inches).

It is very reassuring when this examination confirms that your baby is healthy. If any problem is identified, it can be dealt with quickly.

The heel prick test

The heel prick test is performed on all newborn babies. It is a screening test that detects six serious disorders all of which can be treated successfully if picked up quickly after birth. The most common ones are cystic fibrosis (1 in 1500), hypothyroidism (1 in 3000) and phenylketonuria (PKU) (1 in 7000). The other three are homocystinuria, maple-syrup urine disease and galactosaemia. (The test establishes whether your baby is able to process the protein and carbohydrate in the milk he or she is being fed.) The process involves taking a sample of blood from the baby's heel. The timing of the sample is critical. The blood is obtained on day 4 if the baby is bottle-fed and day 5 if breastfed. At this stage most mothers and babies have returned home. You may bring your baby back to the hospital to have the test done or your public health nurse may call to your home to do it.

A small amount of blood is obtained from your baby's heel using a lancet. The blood is absorbed on to a specially designed card which is then sent to the central metabolic screening laboratory. There it is tested immediately and if there is any abnormality the hospital and your GP will be contacted urgently so that treatment can begin at once.

Vitamin K

Vitamin K will be given to your baby soon after birth. This is a substance which is necessary for normal blood clotting. If levels are too low, the baby is prone to develop the bleeding condition 'haemorrhagic disease of the newborn'. For this reason it is current policy to administer vitamin K to all infants. It is given by injection to all babies within 24 hours of birth. Because breast milk is low in vitamin K breastfed babies are given further doses, orally, on day 4, at one month old and then monthly until the baby is weaned off the breast. Vitamin K is contained in baby milk formulae.

Umbilical cord (belly button) care

At birth a clamp is placed on your baby's umbilical cord close to where it enters the tummy and the remainder is cut. This remaining stump quickly involutes (shrivels) and the clamp is removed on the second or third day. The remaining piece of the cord continues to shrivel and it will separate away completely by the end of the first week. The nurses will show you how to care for the cord by cleaning it with cotton wool and water. The use of antibiotic powders is no longer recommended as they delay the natural shrivelling and separation process.

Common conditions in newborn babies
Jaundice
Jaundice is a yellow discolouration of the skin and is commonly seen in newborn babies. It is due to a yellow substance called bilirubin which is formed from the natural breakdown of red blood cells. This bilirubin is handled and disposed of by the liver. In newborn babies the liver is sluggish and the bilirubin collects in the blood. In most cases the jaundice is harmless and it settles in a matter of a few days.

However, on rare occasions excessively high levels can cause deafness and a variety of cerebral palsy. If there is a suspicion of jaundice, a sample of blood will be taken to check the level. If the level is high, your baby will be treated by phototherapy which helps to eliminate the jaundice from the body. This is a simple, safe technique. A special ultraviolet lamp is placed over the baby, who is unclothed apart from a nappy. The treatment usually takes 24–48 hours.

Sticky eyes (conjunctivitis)
Sticky eyes, or conjunctivitis, is very common in the first few days after birth. A newborn baby produces very few tears. In the absence of tears the eye is prone to infection because tears have irrigation and antiseptic properties. The infection is usually mild and is treated by cleaning with cotton wool and water. If the infection is severe or persistent the doctor will prescribe topical eye drops or ointment.

Sometimes the eye infection is due to a blocked tear duct. While this not a serious problem, it means that the eye will remain sticky intermittently over a period of a few weeks until the duct opens up. You should clean the eye with cotton wool and water and gently massage the duct opening. You will be shown how to do this.

Thrush
Thrush is a white coating on the baby's tongue and the inside of the cheeks. It is not serious or painful and does not interfere with feeding. It should not be confused with the slight white discolouration of the tongue which is simply due to the fat in the milk. Thrush is easily treated with Mycostatin suspension or Daktarin gel.

Thrush can also cause a nappy rash. The rash is dull red in appearance with small broken areas of skin. Mycostatin or Daktarin are effective treatments.

Naming and registering your baby
Your baby's birth and names, both given and surname, must be registered within three months of the birth. This service is provided by the hospital. If your baby is not registered while you are in hospital you will need to go to your local registration office.

Some parents choose a first name during the pregnancy while others wait until after the birth. Younger mothers tend to have a name ready while older women wait until they see what the baby looks like. Many mothers and fathers agonise for days before making a decision. The process is probably not helped by the bewildering choice of names on offer in the many publications on the subject. Although it can sound like a big task, it is usually not too important in the long term. The name quickly becomes identified with your baby. Most children are happy with their names.

The more important question is the surname. If you are single you may be uncertain as to whether to register your own surname or that of your baby's father. You should discuss the matter during the pregnancy as the time after the birth is very busy. Remember that once your baby's surname has been registered it cannot be changed.

Breastfeeding your baby

Feeding your baby is the single biggest task facing you. You will probably have decided before the birth whether to breast- or bottle-feed. The advantages and disadvantages of the two methods of feeding are widely discussed in hospital antenatal classes, women's magazines, books on the care of the infant and health promotion literature.

There is an abundance of scientific evidence to show that breastfeeding is far superior to bottle feeding. You should therefore make every effort to breastfeed. In Scandinavian countries more than 90 per cent of mothers breastfeed so there is no reason why you shouldn't too. While it may be difficult in the beginning, the midwives in the hospital will help you as best they can and after you go home there is support available in the community. All mothers, but especially those who have had a forceps or caesarean delivery, need help at this time. With pressure on beds in the Irish hospital system you may be discharged home before feeding is fully established and this may create difficulties for you. Remember the voluntary support agencies (see panel) which provide help, either over the phone or in your own home.

You need practical help and advice on how to get your baby to latch on properly. See panel *How to breastfeed*. This is very important as the baby's sucking stimulates milk production and if the stimulus is inadequate not enough milk will be produced. Incorrect positioning can lead to cracked nipples which become painful when the breasts become engorged with milk on the third day. The baby's lips should be on the brown area around the nipple (areola). If there are early

how to breastfeed

Make skin contact with your baby as early as possible, preferably in the delivery ward immediately after the birth.

Put your baby to the breast as soon as practical after the birth, again preferably in the delivery ward.

Hold your baby so that he or she is comfortable, with the body well supported and the head in the crook of your elbow facing your breast.

Put your baby's mouth at the same level as your breast.

Bring your baby to your breast, not your breast to your baby, and brush your nipple lightly against the baby's lips. The baby's mouth should open reflexively; when it is wide open let the baby take the breast in the mouth. The nipple should be far back in the mouth and the nose should be touching the breast.

Relax and enjoy the sensation. Breastfeeding is a wonderful time to enjoy eye contact with your new baby—in the early weeks a baby's eyes focus best at breast—eye distance—and for you to get to know each other better.

Position your baby correctly to help prevent, and heal, sore nipples.

difficulties milk can be expressed with a milk pump and then fed to your baby. In some situations where the amount of breast milk is insufficient, it can be supplemented with top up artificial feeds until feeding is fully established. It can take two or three days to get breastfeeding going and it can take two to three weeks to get it fully established. Patience and persistence are very important.

Common problems with breastfeeding

The baby may not latch on properly to your breast or may be drowsy and continually fall asleep at the breast. Jaundice may develop although it is rarely severe enough to require treatment. It may cause your baby to be a little sleepy. A forceps or vacuum delivery may make your baby a bit irritable or out of sorts. Babies born before term at 38 weeks or less tend to be slow feeders. Sometimes, otherwise completely normal babies are poor breastfeeders. Your nipples may become sore and cracked. Good nursing support in the first days after birth can prevent most of these problems. The days of sore nipples, a sore perineum and a constantly crying baby are now uncommon.

In the event of sore nipples, check that the positioning is correct. The important points here are to ensure that the baby's mouth is wide open before the breast is taken, that the areola (the dark-skinned part around the nipple) and not just the nipple is taken into the mouth, and that the baby is close to you so that the lips and chin are touching your breast. Avoid using nipple shields, they don't help and almost always reduce your milk supply. Bottles and soothers can cause 'nipple confusion', which will make your baby suck differently and thereby cause your nipples to become painful. Rub a little of the breast milk onto your nipples as this will help soothe them. Avoid using anything on your nipples, other than water or breast milk unless prescribed by a doctor or advised by a midwife or lactation consultant. If your breasts are too sore to continue feeding you should try expressing milk and feeding it to your baby with a spoon or cup until your breasts have recovered. Avoid using a bottle as this can cause nipple confusion. If you are still in hospital the midwives will help you to express milk, otherwise you can contact one of the support groups.

The nature of breast milk

Breast milk production is a dynamic process. The composition and volume of milk changes rapidly in the early days after birth. The small amount of concentrated milk produced in the first 48 hours is called colostrum and contains many ingredients to promote and develop your baby's defences against infection. From the third day the volume of breast milk begins to increase and its composition alters to that of mature milk. When breastfeeding is fully established towards the end of the first week, a full breast contains 90 ml (3 fl oz). There is a consistent average milk production of 800 ml of breast milk per 24 hours. Once this ceiling has been reached it is unlikely that the production of milk can be increased.

The changing nature of breast milk content continues over the whole period of breastfeeding. If you are overworked or overtired, the fat content in your milk tends to diminish leading to a reduction in calories. Breast milk produced by mothers of premature babies is significantly different in composition and uniquely adapted to the special needs of a low birth-weight infant.

A baby obtains most of the milk in a breast in the first six minutes of the feed. You will rapidly learn how to tell that a feed is completed as the breasts will feel lighter. Continued suckling after this time has more comforting and sedative than nutritive value. Sometimes your baby will be satisfied with one breast and then fall asleep but usually will feed from both breasts.

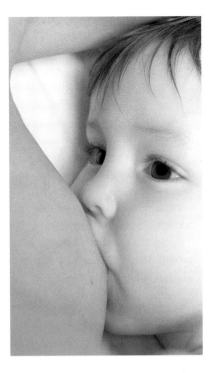

Is my baby getting enough milk?

While breastfeeding usually progresses very well once it is established, it does require supervision and monitoring. The fact that your baby appears satisfied, cries little and seems contented cannot always be relied on as a sign that all is well as some breastfed babies who are undernourished do not cry or demand more. Useful clues to under-feeding are cold hands and feet and loose skin over the inner thighs.

A normal baby gains 180 g (6 oz) per week. Your baby should be weighed every week for 6 weeks so that weight gain can be monitored. This can be arranged through your local health clinic. From time to time your baby may seem hungrier than usual and look for more frequent feeds. This does not mean that he or she is not getting enough but is probably due to a growth spurt. Remember—the more often you give the breast the more milk is produced. Weight gain is the key measure of adequate intake by your baby.

if you are breast-feeding remember

Your baby should be weighed every week for the first six weeks to confirm that feeding is going well

An underfed breastfed baby can appear contented

Your baby gets most of the milk in a breast in the first six minutes

It is safe to take most medications including antibiotics when breast-feeding

Small occasional vomits are normal.

How long should I breastfeed?

You may wonder how long you should continue breastfeeding. There is no right or wrong answer but current advice is to breastfeed until your baby is six months old, the age recommended for starting solids. The decision is up to you and your personal circumstances. Many mothers wean or partially wean their babies at three to four months of age in preparation for returning to work, although it should be possible to continue to breastfeed even after you have returned to work. The ideal is to feed for at least six months so you may wish to extend your maternity leave either by taking unpaid leave or by taking some holiday time. The ease with which you can continue to breastfeed will depend on your circumstances and factors such as availability of crèche facilities at, or close to, work, baby minding facilities and work flexibility, e.g. part time work. You may also wish to express milk and store it at home and a babyminder can give your baby breast milk even if it is from a bottle! So there is a variety of ways in which you can continue to give your baby the benefits of breast milk even after you have returned to work.

cosmetic surgery to the breasts

Cosmetic breast enlargement has now become a more common procedure. If you have had this operation you can still feed your baby as the implant is inserted behind normal breast tissue which is left undamaged.

If you have had a breast reduction operation, however, you cannot breastfeed because the procedure severs the ducts connected to the nipple.

Does it matter if I am taking medication?

If you are taking medication you may be concerned that you are passing it on to your baby through your breast milk and wonder if breastfeeding can be continued. The amount of a medication transmitted through to your breast milk is very small and is most unlikely to affect your baby. Thus commonly used drugs such as antibiotics can be safely taken while you are breastfeeding. However, there are a few exceptions to this rule so it is best to check with your doctor if you are prescribed any medication.

Drinking alcohol

There is varying advice about drinking alcohol while breastfeeding. Again, it appears to be safe if modest amounts are taken. If you drink a glass of wine, the amount that penetrates the breast milk is very small and thus has no impact on your baby.

Bottle-feeding your baby

If you are bottle-feeding your baby, you should start as soon as you reach the postnatal ward. The usual schedule is to feed your baby every four hours.

Milk formulae

There is a wide choice of well-known milk formulae all of which are suitable for your baby. They are based on cow's milk that has been modified to make the protein, fat and carbohydrate more suitable for infants. The correct quantities of vitamins and iron have also been added to the formula.

Soya milk

There are also milk formulae based on soya rather than cow's milk. These milks are used if your baby has cow's milk protein intolerance. However, in recent years they have become less popular because their use increases the risk of developing soya and peanut allergy. You should not start your baby on a soya milk without medical advice.

Goat's milk

Goat's milk is sometimes given to babies with a strong family history of allergies. It is deficient in folic acid. There is now a commercial preparation available with folic acid added. It is generally thought unsuitable for babies.

Heating bottles

Traditionally bottles are heated to body temperature before feeding the baby. There is, however, no need to do this as babies can drink room temperature milk just as well. Heating bottles in a jug can be hazardous because of scalding. Don't use a microwave as it can quickly heat the milk to scalding point in 'hot spots'. Shake the bottle well before feeding. Dedicated bottle heaters are probably best.

Taking your baby home

Most mothers go home two or three days after the birth but if you have had a caesarean section you will need to stay a few days longer. A few mothers opt for an early discharge within 24 hours of birth. Whatever the arrangement, it is important that you feel confident about your baby. In particular you need a definite feeding plan, be it breast, bottle or a combination.

Shortly before leaving, your baby will be weighed. Don't worry about a little weight loss—this is normal and due to your baby getting rid of excess body water. Up to 10 per cent of body weight, which for an average baby is 350 g (11 oz),

bottle-feeding

You will be supplied with made up bottles of feed for your baby. Each bottle contains 100 ml and the average baby will drink approximately 150 ml per kg (2½ fl oz per 1 lb per 24 hours).

For the first week or so after birth babies will feed about 6 times per 24 hours, or once every 4 hours. A hungry baby may not be satisfied and may need a little more. Obviously a baby weighing 4.5 kg (10 lb) will have a bigger appetite!

On the way home you will probably have the opportunity to buy some pre made bottles from the hospital shop, but it is better to organise bottles and a steriliser, and feed, before you go home. Any unused feed has to be thrown out for reasons of hygiene. Instructions with regard to how much to feed your baby are clearly outlined on the food tins that you can buy in any supermarket.

your baby's weight

Your baby will be weighed before going home
Up to 10 per cent weight loss is normal
Your baby will be back to birth weight by day 10

may be lost. After four days the weight loss stops and by day 7–10 birth weight will be regained. After the first ten days there should be a steady weight gain of 180 g (6 oz) per week.

If your baby loses more than 10 per cent of birth weight at the time of leaving hospital your feeding plan will need to be changed. If you are breastfeeding, it may be that your milk is not yet fully established. You will be advised about the best option—to feed more often, express milk with a breast pump or add top up feeds. Whatever the strategy taken, your baby should be weighed again in a matter of a few days.

Before discharge, the umbilical cord will be checked to ensure that it is shrinking and separating properly. Your baby will also be examined to check that there is nothing amiss and that he or she seems contented.

If you are taking your baby home in a car you should use a suitable, correctly fitted car seat. Do not place your baby in the front seat if the car has an air bag on the passenger side.

small vomits or possets

Small vomits or possets are common and the amount of milk involved is rarely significant. These little vomits can be reduced by keeping your baby upright after feeds. It takes 90 minutes for a baby's stomach to empty.

The early days at home

The first few days at home with a new baby, particularly if it is your first, are tinged with a mixture of excitement and anxiety. You may be worried about feeding and sleeping problems and your general ability to cope. Irrespective of your previous experience and support arrangements, there are a few basic rules that will stand you in good stead.

All babies have the same pattern of activity—sleeping, gradually waking up, crying for a feed, being alert and playful, followed by a further period of sleeping. The problem is that individual babies spend variable amounts of time at each of these activities.

When crying predominates over sleeping, parents quickly become worried, drained and exhausted. From the medical viewpoint, the important issue is whether the baby is well or ill. If he or she is feeding well and keeping the milk down, this is reassuring. The nature of the cry is helpful. Healthy babies have a loud vigorous cry, sick babies have a more low-pitched whimper. Healthy babies have a pink colour, sick babies have a poor greyish colour. Trust your instincts. If your baby is out of sorts and different to previously, call the doctor.

During the first week you will quickly get to know your new baby. All babies have their own individual likes and dislikes—personality starts on day one. A baby will prefer to be held in a certain way, fed in a certain way, played with at certain times, left to settle at other times. These preferences are part of the emerging persona and should be given due note and respect.

Your new-born baby has a vast array of non-verbal skills which will be used to constantly communicate with you. Examples include eye contact, facial expressions and a variety of body movements. If you quickly study and learn these signals, it will greatly increase your confidence in handling and understanding your baby. Like you the baby is also learning. Babies quickly grasp the feeding routine and hopefully the difference between day and night! Within days your baby will recognise your face and voice and when you make faces will try to copy you. Your baby will make little noises to attract your attention and will stare intently at you. You will probably be able to detect a smile from three weeks onwards.

Why your baby cries

A crying baby is giving a signal that something is wrong. Your baby cries for a variety of reasons, some important, some trivial. The common, easy to sort causes are hunger, discomfort from a nappy that needs changing, wind or colic, boredom, loneliness. The problem arises when you have attended to all these tasks but the crying continues.

For decades books about baby care have discussed whether babies should be picked up when they cry. The current advice is to pick up as soon as crying starts. Leaving a baby to cry only increases feelings of isolation and erodes self-confidence. There is good evidence that babies who are tended to quickly ultimately cry less. Babies are never manipulative: they only cry when they want help. They do not try to control or be assertive, they simply want to be looked after. The notion that babies who are picked up will be 'spoiled' is not correct.

Colic

Colic is a term used for episodes of loud crying during which the baby appears to be in pain. This uncontrolled and excessive crying begins in the first few weeks in some healthy babies. No-one really knows what causes it but it is not due to hunger or wind and is rarely due to cow's milk intolerance. It is, however, often confused with wind, a condition that can be managed by correct winding during and after feeding.

There are a variety of 'over the counter' preparations designed to alleviate the problem of colic but it is debatable how effective they are. Lactaid drops can be added to bottle-feeds. These drops break down the lactose in the milk and it is hoped that this will prevent excess fermentation and gas production. Infacol drops, which can be given to both breast and bottle-fed infants, help to reduce the collection of wind.

drowsy babies

In the first few days after birth your baby may be drowsy and slow to wake up. Any drowsy baby should be examined to make sure that all is well. Usually all that is necessary is to wait until the baby gets going which happens over a period of 48 hours. During this time it is best to wake the baby every four hours and offer a feed. Waking should be done gently, there is no need to rush. As the eyes open, roll the baby over and loosen the blankets. If sleepiness persists try changing the nappy.

If your baby has colic you and your partner will quickly become exhausted, particularly if you are being woken frequently at night. A healthy baby's cry can be very intense reaching 60 to 70 decibels. If your baby is going through a crying patch you will need support and help. You will feel better if you get a little break for a few hours while someone else minds your baby.

If the crying is getting difficult and unmanageable, seek medical advice. Don't accept the unhelpful comment 'we all had to put with it'. Some babies with excessive crying have reflux and respond well to medication. Usually the crying peaks at four to six weeks and then gradually improves. If it is not settled by three months, medical intervention with investigations and treatment should be considered.

How to recognise when your baby is sick and what to do

All parents worry about their baby getting sick. What are the signs? What do you look for? How do you distinguish between a minor problem and a serious illness. What do you do, who do you contact?

A simple rule of thumb is that any baby who is out of sorts should be considered sick. The first sign is often a change in the pattern of feeding, settling and waking. The baby may feel hot with a raised temperature. However, the absence of fever in a small baby does not mean they don't have an infection.

Sick babies feed poorly: you should be concerned if milk intake decreases by more than one third. Vomiting, when persistent, is another concern. The nappies may be dry because of poor urine output, or there may be diarrhoea. Poor colour and rapid breathing are important signs that all is not well. Irritability, which is an important early feature of meningitis, is difficult to describe and definition is somewhat subjective. A baby can be considered irritable if a straightforward procedure such as changing a nappy or a babygro now causes distress, shown by crying. A sick baby is difficult to console and continues to cry despite your best efforts.

If your concerns about your baby persist for more than four to six hours, it is likely that something is wrong. You need to see a doctor to try to find out what the matter is. Babies get sick more quickly than older children and adults. Have a plan about how you will get medical help in the event of your baby becoming sick. The options are to visit your GP's surgery, to ask your GP to make a home visit, to go back to the hospital where you gave birth if the baby is less than 6 weeks old, or if the baby is over 6 weeks to go to the nearest hospital with a children's unit.

Quite often the doctor will not have an immediate diagnosis. The first task is to decide whether the baby is mildly unwell or seriously sick. Even if the illness is thought to be minor, you must remain vigilant and get your baby reviewed if there is no improvement within 24 hours. In a small baby irritability, fever and poor feeding can be indicative of a variety of conditions and the correct diagnosis can only be reached after a series of laboratory and x-ray investigations.

Vaccinations

Vaccination is a cornerstone of good childcare. It offers the promise of a healthier childhood. The young baby will be better protected when in contact with other individuals, particularly if attending a crèche. The older child is better equipped to deal with the greater exposure to infection at school entry.

The current schedule protects a child from twelve diseases. It is likely that the schedule will be added to in the future.

The vaccination programme is carefully set out in terms of timing of the various shots. In the Dublin area the BCG vaccine, which protects against tuberculosis is administered shortly after birth, it is given at a later stage in other parts of the country. BCG leaves two marks on the left upper arm, which subsequently crust over before clearing to two small marks.

Side effects of the other vaccinations, if any, are minor: they consist of a slight temperature or a little soreness at the site of the injection.

Vaccination is strongly recommended. You need to give considerable thought to a decision not to vaccinate your baby against a specific condition. Failure to vaccinate leaves a baby completely exposed to that disease and its complications. Busy modern lifestyles expose babies to infection at an earlier age.

schedule of vaccinations

At birth: BCG (tuberculosis)
At 2 months: 6 in 1 (diphtheria, tetanus, whooping cough, Hib (haemophilus influenzae B), polio, Hepatitis B), PCV (pneumoococcal conjugate vaccine)
At 4 months: 6 in 1, Men C (meningococcal C)
At 6 months: 6 in 1, Men C, PCV
At 12 months: MMR (measles, mumps, rubella), PCV
At 13 months: Men C, Hib

Choosing childcare

A high proportion of mothers in Ireland return to work when their babies are three to six months old. In preparation for this return to the workforce, childcare options have to be considered. Some mothers are lucky to have a relative who can step in, most don't. You may have a minder in your own home, have your baby minded with another family, or in a crèche.

Crèches

More babies are now looked after in crèches as individual childcare has become scarce and expensive.

When choosing a crèche there are a number of important points to consider. One is proximity: it is a great advantage to have the crèche nearby, particularly in a congested city like Dublin. The crèche should be clean and organised. It should have three or four separate rooms, a kitchen for making up bottles and feeds, toilet/bathroom, playroom, sleeping area, and an outdoor facility for toddlers and older children. Babies and toddlers must be physically separated.

The recommended guidelines for space per baby according to age are:
- Under 1 year: 3.7 sq metres
- 1–2 years: 2.8 sq metres
- Over 2 years: 2.3 sq metres.

Go into every room when you are inspecting a crèche. See what general baby equipment is available—high chairs, nappy changing area, sleeping facilities. What are the fire safety precautions? How many members of staff are there? Babies need more carers than older children, they are completely dependant on adults for everything. They should be looked after separately from older children.

The recommended staff ratios are:
- Under 1 year: 1 adult to 3 babies
- 1–3 years: 1 adult to 6 children
- 3–6 years: 1 adult to 8 children.

Ask about the qualifications of the staff. Find out how bottles and food are prepared and note the level of hygiene. Ask how the day is organised in relation to feeding, sleeping, playing and individual needs. Ask staff what they do when a baby cries between feeds. Babies must always be held when feeding and never fed from a propped up bottle. Be sure you understand what the crèche's procedures are if your baby becomes ill. The crèche must have good phone communications so that you can ring about your baby at any time.

choosing a childminder

You should formally interview a potential childminder.
She must like babies.
Check the childminder's references.
Specify how you want your baby looked after.
After one week you will know whether the arrangement is working.

Childminder

Selecting a minder to look after your baby at home needs to follow a set format. First and foremost you must like the individual, she will be in your house every day looking after your baby. She will know a lot about you and your private life. Find out about her previous experience with small babies. Somebody who has applied because she couldn't get a job at anything else is not suitable. Ask her how she would set about minding your baby and the schedule she would put in place.

Some parents make the mistake of expecting their baby minder to do large amounts of household chores as well as caring for their baby. Be clear: do you want a baby minder or a housekeeper? They are two separate jobs and you are not going to get one individual to do both.

References are essential and you must contact at least one of the referees by phone. When you have employed a new minder, you should drop home during the day to check that all is well. Be sensitive and aware of any changes in your baby's behaviour which could be a sign that the care is inadequate.

Travel and holidays

Many families ask about whether it is advisable to take babies and small children abroad. Clearly where you intend going is relevant. The more distant the destination, the more likely that medical services will be difficult to assess. When taking a baby away, always have a plan about what to do if an illness develops. You should explore the issue of medical care and facilities with the travel agent before you get on the plane.

One of the commonest risks is gastroenteritis. If you are bottle-feeding, you must pay great attention to washing bottles and making up feeds. You should use bottled water and boil it before use.

The plane journey is less of a hazard. Your baby may experience some ear pain on descent; this can be alleviated by giving a feed at that time.

Long car journeys can be a problem. Many young children become miserable if they have to endure trips lasting longer than one or two hours. In the case of longer journeys, you should make regular stops.

In hot climates, and even in Ireland, sunburn is a real risk and it can happen quickly. Babies placed in the shade can end up exposed to full sun in a matter of an hour or two. Small babies should mostly be kept indoors. When taking your baby out in the sun, apply factor 15 sun cream and a bonnet.

Developmental milestones

Development is the process of unfolding, expanding, becoming more complex and more complete. By its very nature it is a slow process. Each baby develops in his or her own individual way.

A baby's development starts at the head and works downwards. The pace differs between babies but the sequence is always the same.

the six-week check-up

It is usual and advisable for babies to have a medical check-up at six weeks. You can bring your baby to your GP, the maternity hospital or to your local health clinic, whichever is most convenient. This is a good age at which to assess how your baby has been doing. Any problems can be discussed and sorted out. Your baby will be weighed and measured. At six weeks the weight will be at least 1 kg (2.2 lb) above birth weight, length will be 5 cm (2 inches) longer, the head will be 5 cm (2 inches) bigger. The first six weeks is the period of most rapid growth in life.

Babies look bigger and more robust at this stage and their little arms and thighs have filled out because this is where they lay down fat as they grow.

During the first six weeks babies develop many new tricks. They smile readily and watch and follow objects. Head control is now much better. They are able to bear weight on their legs and they make little noises to attract attention. Their hands are open and make frequent wriggling movements.

Babies are aware of their surroundings from birth. They can see faces at short distances and will look at you intently when feeding. Hearing is well developed from birth and loud sounds will startle a newborn baby. However, babies can't locate a sound source, they do not turn their heads to noises until after seven months.

Eye contact is the earliest sign of babies' development, it is present almost immediately after birth. It is their method of communication, they are good non-verbal communicators. Facial expression and frowning quickly follow. The first social smiles appear at three weeks. Vocalisation and following you with their eyes are well established at six weeks. In these early weeks and months babies are only interested in faces and voices. They have only a passing interest in toys and mobiles. There are new changes every day as your baby quickly gets bigger and stronger.

By three months there will be good head control. The next milestone is to start looking at and then using the hands. Sitting is a big skill and takes a baby a few months to perfect. It is usually well established by nine months. The next motor stage is crawling, followed by walking at 15 months.

Parents are often concerned when a baby is not able to perform a specific skill. This is usually just a variation of normal. Babies with a problem have global delay, in other words they are behind in all facets of development. If you are at all concerned about your baby's development contact your GP in the first instance.

When to introduce solid food

It is easy to understand that the stomach of a young baby is only designed for milk. The question is when the older baby is capable of digesting solid food. This has been a matter of debate for years. The current thinking is that six months is the right age to introduce solids. There must, however, be some latitude. Some babies can become very hungry and need solids a little sooner. The starter food is also important. Baby rice is the recommended first food, being an easy to digest carbohydrate. To begin with, you should give enough to cover the tip of a flat plastic spoon and build up over a short period to three spoon feeds a day.

When feeding has been established on baby rice, you can start experimenting with other foods. Fruit purees are popular and there is a wide range. Later, after six months, you can give cereals and yogurt. You can liquidise most of your home cooked foods as long as it is not fried and does not contain added salt or sugar. Many babies like mashed banana. Mashed potato is another common and tasty food. Like adults, babies quickly develop likes and dislikes and you will understand this when your baby starts refusing, spitting back or vomiting certain foods.

introducing solid foods

Delay solids until six months

Rice is the best starter food

If giving home-cooked food, don't give fries and do not add salt or sugar

Don't feed your baby tin or packet soups

Avoid egg and wheat products in the first six months

Salt must not be added to food as young kidneys have difficulty in eliminating excess salt. Similarly, tinned and packet soups should not be given because of their salt content. Fruit juices are no longer advisable, as the acidity may damage the enamel on emerging teeth.

Some foods are more likely to cause an allergic reaction. Eggs are best avoided in the first six months. Other foods with an allergic potential include tomatoes, strawberries and peanut butter. Allergy to peanuts has become more frequent, probably because peanut oil is included in so many food preparations nowadays. So try to keep your baby's diet simple and avoid exotic foods.

Frequently asked questions

When can babies see?
Babies can see from birth. They quickly recognise their parents, by three weeks will be smiling at them, by six weeks will be watching and following objects.

By what age will my baby's eyes change colour?
By four months. All babies have blue eyes at birth but if they inherit brown eyes, the colour will change by four months.

Sometimes when my baby is asleep his eyes roll and he appears restless. Why is this?
This is rapid eye movement (REM) sleep, also known as dream sleep. It accounts for about 50 per cent of small babies' sleep. During REM they process the day's experience.

There is a red mark in the middle of my baby's forehead—will it go?
Yes, it will disappear. A red mark in the centre of the forehead and the eyelids is very common. It is called a 'stork bite' or 'salmon patch'. It is due to a minor imbalance in the blood supply to the skin and it resolves as the skin matures.

There is a blue spot on my baby's back. What is this and will it go?
Dark skinned babies frequently have a blue spot on the back or buttocks and all Asian babies have it—it is quite normal. The spot fades with time.

What are strawberry marks?
These are pink lumps on the skin, usually the trunk. There is usually only one. They are not present at birth, but develop shortly afterwards and are more common in premature babies and girls. They should not be treated as they gradually go white and shrink, and finally disappear after about three years.

My baby has a scaly rash on her eyebrows and cheeks. What is this?
This is seborrhoec dermatitis, a temporary, harmless rash. It is not eczema. It does not weep or crust and your baby does not scratch it. It should be treated with emulsifying ointment. If it is persistent, the doctor will prescribe a dilute hydrocortisone ointment.

My baby is snuffly: what should I do?

This is common and is not caused by an infection or a cold. The best remedy is to keep the baby upright after feeds. This allows any mucus present to drain away.

My baby has a nappy rash: what should I do about it?

Nappy rashes have become uncommon since the advent of the disposable nappy. Minor rashes will respond to a barrier cream. If the rash is dull red with irregular edges it is thrush. This is easily treated with Mycostatin or Daktarin ointment.

The back of my baby's head looks flat—should I be concerned?

No. This is very common—it is caused by the baby lying on her back. It will correct itself as she gets older.

My baby tilts her head to one side. Why is this?

Some babies prefer to turn their head to either the left or right. This results in a tilted appearance which can be corrected by simple measures. Encourage her to turn the other way, e.g. if she tends to turn to the right, you can get her to turn left by feeding her placed on your right arm. Talk to her from the left side and place toys on the left side. If she persists in turning one way, a paediatric physiotherapist will give additional exercises.

The soft spot is still present. Is this normal?

The soft area on the top of the baby's head, the anterior fontanelle, allows the skull bones to expand as the brain grows. It is present until the baby is over 18 months old.

My baby's breasts look swollen. Is this normal?

Yes. Both girls and boys have swollen breasts at birth. It is due to the action of the mother's hormones during the pregnancy. The swellings will recede spontaneously. Under no circumstances squeeze the breasts as this can cause infection.

Should my baby boy be circumcised?

The simple answer is no. It would be of no benefit to your baby, would cause him pain and can result in complications such as infection and bleeding. It is an unnecessary procedure and is not recommended by paediatricians.

When can we take our baby boy swimming?

It is perhaps best to wait until he is three or four months old. Very young babies have difficulty in maintaining their body temperature and so are likely to get cold. Until your baby is four months old he will have poor head control which will make it difficult to hold him properly in the water. Also, bringing him into contact with many other children at a young age would expose him to the risk of infection such as gastroenteritis.

Is it safe for my baby to fly?

It is safe to fly at a young age. Your baby may get ear pain on descent which can be alleviated by feeding. As with all travel the main risk for babies is picking up an infection. Stick to your established routines of feeding and changing. Don't let him get overtired.

Sometimes my baby's stools are green—does this matter?

The colour of a healthy baby's stool is quite variable. It depends on how long the stool has been formed before it is passed. It goes through a series of colours from yellow to brown and then to green.

My baby passes lots of wind—should I be concerned?

This is perfectly normal. Babies' bowels are very active particularly when they are breastfed. The passing of wind is simply part of this normal bowel activity.

What can I give my baby for constipation?

Ask advice before giving your baby anything—she may not be constipated. It is quite normal for her to have a bowel motion only every two or three days as long as the motion is not hard. If the motions are hard, they can be softened with cooled boiled water between bottle feeds or a sugar-based laxative such as Duphalac.

There is a discharge from my baby's belly button. What should I do?

This condition is called an umbilical granuloma. It is a small piece of the umbilical cord that has not detached. It is easily treated by your GP. A piece of silver nitrate is applied which helps it to shrink.

My baby's belly looks large. Is that normal?

Yes, all babies have large, floppy bellies. They have not yet developed their abdominal muscles. Babies start to develop their tummy muscles when they start trying to sit up.

When will my baby sleep through the night?

The age at which babies stop waking for a feed at night varies. They tend to settle after three months. At that stage they are taking larger feeds and can thus last a bit longer.

When do children talk?

The development of speech is a gradual, steady process. Babies start to 'coo' at about six weeks. Over the subsequent months they become more vocal and this is followed by a period of babbling. At 18 months babies have single words, by two years they are be able to put three-word sentences together.

What should I do to prevent cot death?

Cot death has become less common over the last decade. Avoid cigarette smoking. Put the baby to sleep on her back—the 'back to sleep' advice. Don't let her become over heated. If you take her into your bed, be careful not to fall asleep and lie on top of her.

I've been told my baby has tongue tie and needs an operation to fix it. Is this true?

There is a piece of tissue under the tongue attached to the floor of the month. Very occasionally it is short and tight. It may sometimes cause difficulties with breast feeding and may need to be divided. If your baby is feeding without difficulty it doesn't need to be divided.

abcess An abcess is a fluid collection of infectious material (pus), which can occur in the breast in association with breastfeeding or in a wound, usually following caesarean delivery. Symptoms include fever and redness, swelling and exquisite tenderness in the affected area. Breast abcess is usually the result of untreated mastitis. Although agonising, it is important for you to continue feeding the baby or expressing milk right through the infection to keep the breast empty and free of blocked milk ducts. If you develop an abcess, treatment is by incision and drainage under general anaesthesia. A wound abcess may drain itself spontaneously.

'My mastitis came on really fast one evening when Sam was four weeks old. First it felt like there was something rubbing at the side of my breast, like a seam from my bra. Then I started to feel a bit tired and fluey. Within three hours I had a fever and my breast had begun to ache. I got straight into a hot bath for a few hours thinking I had a blocked duct or something and that the bath might ease the milk out, meanwhile I fed on the healthy side. By the next morning I was in absolute agony— leaking and engorged on the sore side, with a really high fever and aching all over. The doctor came round and said I had mastitis and an abcess, probably from an infection creeping in through a slightly cracked nipple. I went straight in to hospital and had it drained and started a heavy duty course of antibiotics. Luckily, I had plenty of milk in the freezer to tide the baby over while I was gone and I was able to start feeding again when I got home. I was nervous about continuing to breastfeed initially but didn't want to give up. Thankfully, I didn't have any more problems feeding the baby or my subsequent children.'

abdominal pain/tummy pain. It is important to distinguish between discomfort and pain. Discomfort, and even some mild pain, are normal in pregnancy. Most of the causes of abdominal pain during pregnancy are of no medical significance. Only severe abdominal pain, which limits your movement and is accompanied by other symptoms like vomiting, fever or bleeding, needs urgent medical attention. Cramping pains in your uterus are normal in early pregnancy and are often referred to as 'growing pains'.

abnormality (*see* **congenital abnormality**)

abortion (*see also* **termination**) This is the medical term for a pregnancy that ends before 24 weeks. It is also known as miscarriage. Abortion may be spontaneous or induced (termination of pregnancy). Complete abortion occurs when the contents of the uterus are passed with no tissue left behind. Incomplete abortion usually requires curettage (the 'c' part of d&c)to empty the uterus. Missed abortion refers to the death of the foetus with no passing of tissue and usually requires a d&c. Septic abortion occurs when infection is present, as can happen with an intrauterine contraceptive device (IUCD). Threatened abortion is the term used when any vaginal bleeding occurs before 12 weeks. Any bleeding in pregnancy should be investigated—the simplest way to see that the baby is safe in early pregnancy is by ultrasound.

abruptio placentae Abrupt separation of the normally situated placenta. It is an uncommon condition where part or all of the placenta separates prematurely, that is before the baby is delivered. It is often associated with bleeding, but not always because volumes of blood can be lost directly into the uterus without being noticed. This condition may cause sudden death of the baby.

acetone The chemical substance in urine and breath, associated with dehydration, for example with excessive vomiting in early pregnancy. High levels may require intravenous fluids for correction.

active management of labour A sensitive approach to the care of women in their first labours, which involves comprehensive antenatal education, the assignment of one personal midwife to the woman in labour, encouragement to attend the hospital early in labour, early breaking of the waters and administration of oxytocin if the labour is not progressing. This approach is associated with a lower rate of forceps and caesarean delivery and its success appears to be uninfluenced by liberal use of epidurals for pain relief. It is effectively the 'birth plan' of the National Maternity Hospital for first-time mothers although the principles are applicable to all labours.

afterbirth (*see* **placenta**)

afterpains Painful uterine contractions occurring after the baby is born. Following birth, the uterus continues to contract dramatically so that it may return to its normal size. Initially, these contractions can be uncomfortable at the least. The pain varies from mild period-like cramps for first time mothers to very strong pains that make second and third time mothers double over and require pain relief in the days immediately following the birth. The pain should only persist for the first few days after the baby is born and may be felt more acutely during breastfeeding. Bleeding may also intensify during the contractions.

AIDS (*see* **HIV**)

air travel is generally safe in a pregnancy that is proceeding without complications. It does not cause miscarriage or have any effect on a pregnancy. However, most airlines are reluctant to allow travel beyond 34 weeks and some will refuse to carry you beyond 32 weeks in case you go into labour. Likewise, most do not allow staff who are pregnant to fly. If you are on a long flight, keep well hydrated and exercise your leg muscles every hour by walking and flexing your feet. Both measures will help prevent clots forming in your legs, which is an increased risk in pregnancy whether on the ground or in the air. Once you are noticeably pregnant you should get a note from your doctor to say it is safe for you to fly just in case you are questioned at check-in.

alpha fetoprotein (AFP) (*see also* **triple test**) When this protein from the baby's liver is excreted into the amniotic fluid, traces of it enter the maternal circulation. High levels of AFP in a mother's blood are associated with spina bifida and some other rare disorders of the kidney and bowel. High AFP levels alone are not proof of spina bifida—a detailed scan must also be performed to confirm its diagnosis. Likewise, a low level of AFP may be associated with Down syndrome but again is not proof in itself of the condition. AFP comprises only one part of the triple test for Down syndrome.

amenorrhea Absence of periods, most usually caused by pregnancy.

amniocentesis The technique in which a very fine needle is passed through the skin into the amniotic sac to obtain a sample of amniotic fluid for testing—usually used to help detect chromosomal disorders like Down syndrome. It is also used in the management of rhesus disease (blue baby syndrome). Therapeutic amniocentesis is when a large volume of amniotic fluid is drained to relieve pressure symptoms when there is excessive amniotic fluid (polyhydramnios).

amniotic fluid The fluid in the amniotic sac (in which the baby develops) that cushions the baby from shock (*see* **liquor**).

amniotic membrane The membrane, like cling film, that lines the inside of the uterus during pregnancy.

amniotomy Artificial breaking of the waters. The procedure is performed either to induce labour or to visualise the colour and amount of amniotic fluid during labour. The procedure has the effect of shortening the duration of labour if performed after labour has started.

amniotic sac The membrane-lined cavity in which the baby develops.

anal fissure A painful tearing of the back passage associated with childbirth, which causes severe pain on passing a bowel motion and may be accompanied by bleeding. Luckily, it is easily treatable with suppositories supplied on prescription by your doctor. It may very rarely require a small operation.

anaemia If your haemoglobin concentration is less than 10 g/100 ml blood, you have anaemia, usually caused by an iron deficiency. It is normal for the haemoglobin, or iron level to drop during pregnancy because it is diluted by the increase in blood volume but acute reductions should be treated. Having said that, many women mistakenly attribute the characteristic tiredness of early pregnancy to anaemia. Routine blood tests in the early stages of pregnancy will identify problem cases.

anaesthesia (epidural and general) With a general anaesthetic you are fully asleep; with an epidural you will be numb only in the lower part of your body but fully conscious. A spinal anaesthetic is similar to an epidural and is usually given for a caesarean delivery. It works more quickly than an epidural but not for as long.

anencephaly The most severe form of spina bifida, in which the skull and brain fail to develop normally. Anencephaly is fatal—

usually within hours of birth. The condition may be diagnosed by ultrasound as early as 12 weeks. Risk of recurrence is significantly reduced by taking folic acid before you are pregnant and in the early weeks of pregnancy. If your baby has anencephaly, you will be offered counselling and may be referred to a UK clinic for termination if you wish.

antacids Over the counter substances taken to relieve heartburn. Most of them are harmless but you should consult your doctor before taking any medication in pregnancy.

antepartum haemorrhage Any vaginal bleeding that occurs from 24 weeks until delivery is termed an antepartum haemorrhage. The two main causes are placenta praevia and abruptio placentae although there may be local causes as well such as a polyp on the cervix, or neck of the womb. See your doctor if you experience bleeding at any time during your pregnancy.

anteversion The usual, forward leaning position of the uterus in the pelvis (*see* **retroversion**).

anticoagulants Drugs given to thin the blood when there has been a clot in the leg or lung or where there has been a clear history of such a clot in the past. (*see* **Heparin** and **Warfarin**.)

anti D (*see also* **rhesus disease**) A substance that prevents the development of potentially harmful antibodies. It is relevant only to rhesus negative mothers. Blood groups are divided into two broad categories depending on the presence or absence of the rhesus factor. If the rhesus factor is present in your

blood you are rhesus positive, if it is absent you are rhesus negative. Approximately 15 per cent of Irish people are rhesus negative. If you are rhesus negative and some rhesus positive blood enters your bloodstream you will form antibodies against rhesus positive blood. If you are carrying a rhesus positive baby these antibodies may harm your baby by crossing the placenta and causing anaemia. Anti D prevents the development of these antibodies. Risk factors for developing anti rhesus positive antibodies include miscarriage, delivery of a rhesus positive baby, trauma, amniocentesis or chorion villus sampling, external cephalic version and blood transfusion. Anti D prevents the development of rhesus antibodies and will be given to you if any of the risk factors listed above occur. In some countries anti D is given routinely during pregnancy to all rhesus negative women because on rare occasions a baby bleeds into the mother's circulation even though none of the events listed above has occurred.

Apgar score A score reflecting your baby's condition at birth devised by an American anaesthetist, Virginia Apgar. Five criteria are considered: pulse, breathing, colour, movement and response to stimulus. Each function receives a score from 0 to 2, with most babies scoring between 7 and 10. The test is repeated after five to ten minutes. Babies who score poorly initially may require special care at first but even those with a zero score have been known to develop normally.

areola The circular area surrounding the nipple, or areola, will darken and perhaps enlarge in pregnancy. Breastfeeding mothers should aim to get the whole areola into the baby's mouth to prevent cracking the nipples around their base.

arrest of progress When labour proceeds to a certain stage and then stops.

baby blues A temporary feeling of depression, anxiety and irritability in the first week following birth which is completely normal. Changing hormone levels, the shock of birth and new responsibilities conspire to destabilise even the most competent mothers. If these feelings persist for more than a few weeks, they could be symptomatic of more severe post-natal depression and you should consult your GP or hospital. Don't wait until your six week check if you feel you aren't coping or if you feel really low. (*see* **post-natal depression**).

Rachel had an uneventful first pregnancy and was really looking forward to having a baby but she was the first of her friends to have a child and had no family nearby so no one had warned her about how she might feel after the baby arrived. Her whole focus had been on her pregnancy and the birth and she hadn't thought to look beyond them.

'I woke up on the morning of my third day in hospital, turned over to see my new baby asleep in the cot beside me and burst into tears. Looking at her, I suddenly felt I couldn't possibly know or be expected to know how to take care of her. Who on earth could possibly think I was up to this kind of responsibility? What if I failed miserably? I tried to reason with myself

that the hormones were going crazy and made a mental list of all the people I knew who managed to take care of babies and small children. I told myself if they could do it so could I. My partner arrived in the middle of everything and I could tell he was thinking what if she never snaps out of this. I pulled myself together for him but felt pretty rotten for the rest of the day. When my milk came in the panic seemed to ease off although a few times even months later when I was at home the enormity of being completely responsible for another person would hit me like a ton of bricks. It was worst when I was particularly tired and I'd feel very low but I expect every new mother feels like this at some stage.'

backache An extremely common feature of pregnancy, backache is usually due to the loosening of ligaments in your joints because of the relaxing effects of pregnancy hormones. It is usually concentrated in the lower back but in the latter part of pregnancy may also affect the upper part. If the pain becomes severe, your doctor may refer you to a physiotherapist or recommend that you wear a supportive corset brace. Poor posture during breastfeeding may also cause chronic pain. Epidurals do not cause long-term backache.

Bartholins glands Two small glands at the entrance to the vagina that occasionally become blocked and infected although this is unusual in pregnancy.

BCG (Bacille Calmet-Gueret) The vaccine given to newborn babies in many countries, including Ireland, to immunise against tuberculosis. Many hospitals provide the vaccine to babies while they are still in hospital.

Bell's palsy A temporary condition that may arise in pregnancy causing weakness of one side of the face. It can be quite dramatic in appearance but goes away either during pregnancy or soon after delivery.

beta HCG HCG (human chorionic gonadotrophin) is a hormone produced by the developing placenta. Beta HCG is part of HCG. A blood test for beta HCG is usually used to help in diagnosis of ectopic pregnancy and follow up treatment of hydatidiform moles.

bilirubin (*see also* **jaundice**) The yellow chemical formed in the liver from the breakdown of haemoglobin. Excessive amounts cause a yellowing of the skin, or jaundice. Babies whose systems are not yet functioning efficiently may develop jaundice in the days following birth; most babies, particularly breastfed babies, have mild jaundice in the first few days. Jaundice usually disappears on its own but some cases are treated by exposure to ultraviolet (UV) 'bili' lights. The effect of ultra violet light in dissolving bilirubin in the skin was first noticed in a hospital in England. On the post-natal ward there was a balcony where babies were placed on sunny afternoons. It was noticed that the babies' skin remained darkest in the areas least exposed to the sun. Someone put two and two together and deduced that it was the ultraviolet light that was responsible. Hence the development of UV light in the treatment of jaundice of the newborn.

biophysical profile The ultrasound assessment of the health of your baby that may be performed if you are significantly overdue, if your baby is not moving as much as in the past or seems smaller than expected. It measures the amount of amniotic fluid, the baby's movement and muscle tone and whether or not the baby is practising breathing movements. It is scored on a scale of 8, with each category receiving a possible two points. Most scores are between 6 and 8. An additional element in assessment is a foetal heart tracing. If this is used, it is worth another two points. The Doppler flow may also be measured (*see* **Doppler**).

birth plan A wish list of parental preferences for how labour and the birth experience should go (in a perfect world), which can form the basis of discussions with attending doctors and midwives. Whether or not you commit your thoughts to an elaborate document is up to you—the important thing is that you discuss your general preferences about pain relief and care with your partner and professional carers some time before the birth.

birthing chair A device that enables the mother to give birth in an almost upright, gravity-friendly position that has been found to shorten labour slightly. Unfortunately, with it comes an increased risk of postpartum haemorrhage, probably because there is greater congestion of the blood vessels and the design of the chair makes it more difficult to see what is happening. Its use does not lessen the likelihood of forceps deliveries.

bleeding gums During pregnancy, the gums swell and soften making them more susceptible to gum disease and with it, tooth decay. Dentists recommend you make at least one appointment during pregnancy and switch to a softer toothbrush.

blighted ovum An old fashioned term, offensive to many, that describes early miscarriage where the embryo has not developed to the stage where it is visible on ultrasound and has failed to progress from there. The proper term is simply miscarriage.

blood pressure Blood pressure usually drops somewhat in pregnancy but changes in levels are carefully monitored at antenatal visits, particularly as elevated blood pressure is a warning sign of toxaemia. A reading of 140/90 or above is considered high. It is normal to have low blood pressure during pregnancy.

Braxton Hicks' contractions These are 'practice' contractions of the uterus first occurring towards the end of pregnancy (at approximately 35 weeks). They may be quite strong and during a first pregnancy may be confused with the onset of labour. They differ considerably from real labour pains by being less frequent, less persistent, shorter in duration and far less painful. In fact, some women find they are quite pleasant, and feel like nothing more than a superficial but insistent tightening across the belly. Braxton Hicks' contractions are not associated with other possible signs of labour such as a show or rupture of the membranes.

breast care Before birth, no special care of the breasts is needed although you may feel more comfortable in a structured bra. If you are not breastfeeding, in the first few days after the birth you will definitely require a proper nursing bra and your breasts as little stimulation as possible. If you are breastfeeding, keep nipples soft with chamomile cream or lanolin to avoid cracking and change breast pads frequently to avoid germs entering any cracks that do appear. If possible, expose the breasts to both sun and air to help them heal and toughen up faster.

breast pain Your nipples may get very sore while you are pregnant, particularly when it's cold. Warm your breasts up with a hairdryer or take a hot bath to alleviate the pain. As your glands become more active and your pregnancy progresses your breasts may feel quite sore. The growth of the breasts can even strain ligaments and make you feel uncomfortable. Wear a properly fitted maternity bra at all stages of your pregnancy and as long as you feed to give yourself support.

breathlessness Many women find that they are breathless after even minor exertion during all stages of pregnancy. There is no cause for alarm. A sensation of 'catching' your breath is also not unusual and is not a cause for concern either.

breech presentation This describes a baby who is coming out bottom first. About 2 per cent of all babies assume a bottom first position (breech) at the end of pregnancy. Breech presentation is more common in early pregnancy, with the baby frequently turning into the correct position without intervention. It is also more common in women who have been pregnant before. If the baby remains in the breech position, the doctor may try to turn it right way round (external cephalic version) at around week 35–37. If this fails to work, delivery may be by caesarean section.

'On my second pregnancy, the baby felt really, really low from the earliest days. The doctor said she was literally sitting upright towards the end, probably because my uterus was so stretched out from the last baby. Thankfully, she managed to turn herself right way round the night before I was due to go in and have her turned. I didn't think she would because it was so late.'

brow presentation This occurs when the baby's forehead presents against the cervix in labour. It happens when the baby extends his or her neck as if looking upwards. The result is that the diameter of the head presenting in the pelvis is too wide and vaginal delivery is not possible. Delivery has to be by caesarean section with brow presentation.

caesarean section A birth method where the baby is delivered surgically through a cut in the uterus. A lower segment caesarean is the most frequently used procedure where the lower part of the uterus is opened transversely. This is preferable because it is safe to give birth vaginally on subsequent pregnancies. A classical caesarean is when the uterus is opened vertically in the upper part—this is a rare procedure. It is not safe to give birth vaginally after this type of caesarean because there is a significant risk of the uterus rupturing during labour, or

indeed beforehand. A lower segment vertical incision is also sometimes used, particularly in the United States, but opinion is divided on the safety of vaginal birth after this type of caesarean.

caput A collection of fluid on top of a baby's head after delivery. The caput usually disappears within 24 hours of birth.

cardiotocograph (CTG) An electronic tracing of a baby's heart beat is often done during pregnancy to check foetal health, if for example the baby is not moving enough.

carpal tunnel syndrome A collection of symptoms in the hand that include a tingling sensation, weakness and stiffness of the joints. This occurs as a result of fluid retention, which puts pressure on the nerves running into the hand under a band of tissue on the inside of the wrist. Compression of these nerves may cause tingling and numbness in your little finger but may also spread across the hand to other fingers. The condition may be painful and keep you up at night. Your hand may be stiff and sore, in the morning especially. There may also be weakening of the hand muscles, sometimes so pronounced that you may not be able to hold a cup or unscrew a bottle top. Mild carpal tunnel syndrome is common, especially towards the end of pregnancy. The syndrome resolves itself after pregnancy. Surgery to release pressure on the nerves may very rarely be required and braces are available that help ease the symptoms for some people.

caul Part of the amniotic membranes surrounding the baby, which is occasionally stuck to the baby's head like cling film. Historically, being born with a caul, like Oliver Twist, was regarded as bringing good luck.

cephalhematoma If you have a forceps delivery, your baby may be born with a large bruise on top of the head. It will be slower to heal than a caput. It is not harmful.

cephalo-pelvic disproportion *see* **disproportion**

cerebral palsy (CP) An uncommon, progressive condition characterised by stiffening, or spasticity, of movements, for which there is as yet no cure. In 50 per cent of cases physical symptoms are accompanied by a degree of mental retardation. In the past CP was thought to be caused by birth difficulties but now only 10 per cent of cases are felt to be due to difficulties around the time of delivery. The frequency of the condition has not changed in the Western world in the past 30 years.

cervical incompetence A very weak cervix that opens painlessly and is a cause of late miscarriage or very premature delivery. A stitch (cerclage) will be inserted around the cervix in early pregnancy (or, rarely, before pregnancy has begun) if the doctor diagnoses an incompetent cervix. The intention is to prevent late miscarriage or extremely premature delivery (before 24 weeks). Inserting a stitch is a minor procedure performed under general anaesthetic and it is not necessary to stay in hospital after it is performed.

cervix The opening into the uterus, which is made up of fibrous tissue. It shortens (effaces) at the end of pregnancy and dilates (opens) at the beginning of labour. Though not every woman dilates at the same rate or to the same degree, the cervix is considered fully dilated at an average 10 cm.

chickenpox Also known as varicella, chickenpox is a childhood infectious disease which has the potential to damage the baby if contracted in the first 12 weeks of pregnancy or within 4 days before or after the delivery. If you have had chickenpox in the past your baby is protected. A blood test will determine this because antibodies from chickenpox remain in your blood for life. If you are pregnant and less than 13 weeks gestation, and don't know whether or not you have had chickenpox, you should arrange with your doctor to check your immunity. Children with chickenpox are infectious from 48 hours before the rash develops until all of the spots have crusted over. Because chickenpox is so contagious it is likely that any young children who have been exposed to it will catch it. So if you have a toddler in a crèche where there is an outbreak it is likely your child will also get chickenpox. If you are close to delivery then inform your doctor and appropriate protective measures will be arranged to protect your newborn. The major risk for a mother who develops chickenpox in pregnancy is pneumonia so if you get it during pregnancy inform your doctor and be conscious of any respiratory symptoms like a cough.

choriocarcinoma A rare complication of a molar pregnancy (hydatidiform mole) where placental tissue turns malignant. Follow up treatment of a molar pregnancy should ensure that the chances of this happening are reduced.

chorion One of the membranes lining the uterus during pregnancy (see **chorion villus sampling**).

chorion villus sampling (CVS) A technique where a sample of the placenta is taken with a thin needle passed through the cervix via the vagina or through the lower abdomen in early pregnancy for the purpose of diagnosing foetal abnormalities. The baby and the placenta share the same genetic make-up. CVS may be performed later in pregnancy as an alternative to amniocentesis to obtain tissue for chromosomal or chemical analysis. There is an associated risk of miscarriage of approximately 1 per cent.

chromosomes The packages that contain all our genetic material are called chromosomes. There are normally 46 chromosome pairs, with one of each pair inherited from each parent, plus a pair of sex chromosomes: XX in a woman, XY in a man. An extra chromosome, or a rearrangement of part of a chromosome pair, can cause serious problems for a developing baby. An extra chromosome number 21 results in Down syndrome, also known as Trisomy 21. Every ovum (egg) contains one X chromosome, while each sperm contains either an X or a Y chromosome. The sperm therefore is entirely responsible for determining the baby's sex.

circumcision Removal of the foreskin from a baby boy's penis is done primarily for religious reasons and requires general anaesthesia for the baby (in the interests of humanity!). There are virtually no medical reasons for performing it in the newborn period.

cleft or hare lip and palate A congenital malformation of the roof of the mouth and upper lip, which is correctable by surgery. If cleft palate is severe, it may make it difficult for a baby to feed from the breast or a bottle initially and the baby may have to be fed by tube. Surgery for the condition is so good nowadays that virtually no scar is visible afterwards.

clots Collections of blood that have formed a solid lump. Clots are like lumps of jelly when they are forming and then become progressively more firm as they age. A clot several days old may look like a piece of tissue to the inexperienced eye. Passage of clots is not unusual with miscarriage or following delivery. A clot in the leg is more likely to form during pregnancy because the blood is more sticky. A leg clot is charac-terised by pain and swelling of the affected leg, usually below the knee (see **embolus**).

coccyx The bone at the very bottom of the spine. The coccyx may rarely be displaced during labour causing a mother pain after-wards. It generally heals with the passage of time.

colostrum The yellow pre-milk produced by the breasts before birth and for the first few days after birth. It is full of both nourishment and protection against infection.

congenital abnormality Any structural abnormality present from birth. There are a huge number of possible abnormalities including congenital heart disease, kidney abnormalities and conditions like club foot or spina bifida. Some are minor and of almost no significance while others may be life threatening. Approximately 4 per cent of babies have a congenital abnormality and half of these are not serious.

constipation A characteristic feature of pregnancy, due to the relaxing effect of hormones on the bowel muscle, constipation is best prevented by eating a high fibre diet and drinking plenty of fluids. Many women blame the condition on iron supplements, which can intensify the problem. After delivery, it may be a few days before a bowel movement. This is normal and is not to be confused with constipation. As before, if you continue to eat a high fibre diet after the birth, all will be well and you will not need any medication for it.

cordocentesis Passage of a hollow needle through the abdomen and uterus into the umbilical cord close to the placenta or the foetus to obtain a foetal blood sample for testing. This may be done occasionally in cases of rhesus incompatibility, severe chromosome disorders, when specific infections are suspected or if the foetus appears severely growth retarded.

cord prolapse *see* **prolapse (cord)**

corpus luteum That part of the ovary that produces progesterone in the early part of pregnancy. A corpus luteum cyst may form in early pregnancy, but usually disappears spontaneously.

cot death *see* **sudden infant death syndrome**

cotyledon A unit of placental tissue. Occasionally a very adherent cotyledon may remain stuck to the inside of the uterus after delivery. This rarely causes any significant problems but can sometimes lead to infection and abnormally heavy bleeding. It will usually detach itself spontaneously but sometimes a d&c may be necessary.

cramps (abdominal) Tummy pains caused by constipation or contractions are rarely of any significance. Unless they are very severe, persistent or associated with bleeding or a heavy discharge, they are no cause for concern.

cramps (foot and leg) Sharp cramps in the arch of the foot and calf muscles are very common at night and can be extremely painful. Massage and stretch the area until the spasm abates. Taking extra calcium tablets may sometimes prevent them.

cravings It is not unusual to have cravings for certain foods and smells when you are pregnant. Women have been known to crave rubber, coal, ice and even the smell of petrol, not just pickles and ice cream. Avoid eating things that are bad for you no matter how much you want them.

deep vein thrombosis A clot which forms in one of the deep veins, usually in the calf. It causes pain, swelling of one ankle and swollen veins on the surface. The leg itself will also swell and feel tight. The diagnosis is confirmed by measuring the flow of blood in the veins. Treatment is by anti-coagulation drugs. A clot which detaches and travels to another part of the body, usually the lung, is an embolus.

DES (diethylstilbesterol) A hormone that was given to many pregnant women in the past and up until the late 1960s in some countries, under the mistaken impression that it would reduce the chances of miscarriage. Unfortunately, it had no such impact but instead caused significant problems in female offspring. Some experienced an increased incidence of miscarriage themselves, abnormal smears and rarely, cancer of the vagina. It is no longer used.

dilatation The opening of the cervix in labour is measured from a nominal 1 cm to 10 cm. The cervix is considered completely dilated when it can no longer be felt during a pelvic examination.

d&c 'd' refers to the dilatation, or stretching of the cervix, 'c' to the curettage or scraping away of the lining of the womb and emptying of the uterus. In the context of pregnancy, this procedure is used in cases of miscarriage or as a method of termination of pregnancy.

disproportion A rare condition where a baby's head is too large for the pelvis, making it impossible for the head to descend into the pelvis during labour.

dizziness Getting up too fast can make you feel dizzy because of the sudden shifting of blood away from your brain that makes your blood pressure dip (postural hypotension). The solution is simple: always take your time and get up slowly. Dizziness is also common when a meal has been missed and blood sugar levels drop. A quick snack should sort things out. Dizziness may also be caused very occasionally by a disturbance in the middle ear but neither this nor any other dizziness will pose a threat to your baby.

Doppler A form of ultrasound used to measure the speed of blood flow through the baby's blood vessels and umbilical cord. It is often done at the same time as the biophysical profile, usually when the baby appears small for dates or the mother has high blood pressure. It is used to help assess whether the placenta is functioning properly.

doula is Greek for 'handmaiden'. A doula is trained to give emotional and practical support in pregnancy at delivery and after the birth. In Ireland, the personal midwife fulfills the doula role and much more.

Down syndrome A chromosomal abnormality that occurs at the time of conception when the embryo receives an extra chromosome number 21. A baby with Down syndrome has three number 21 chromosomes instead of two. The condition is more common with advancing age of the mother, increasing from 1 in 850 at the age of 30, to 1 in 100 at the age of 40. At 35 the risk is 1 in 350. There is a rare type of Down's that can occur at any age which is due to an abnormality in one parent's chromosomes known as a balanced translocation. This can be diagnosed by performing chromosomal analysis on the parents. Babies with Down syndrome have an increased incidence of other health problems, particularly of the heart and gut, which may require corrective surgery. A varying degree of intellectual disability is inevitable and the milestones of child development (sitting, walking, talking, etc.) will be delayed to a varying degree. Virtually all children with Down's are exceptionally good humoured and pleasant individuals.

Contact Down Syndrome Ireland, tel (01) 873 0999, fax (01) 873 1064, email info@downsyndrome.ie www.downsyndrome.ie

dreams Seriously weird dreams are a characteristic feature of pregnancy and yet another example of the profound effect pregnancy has on the mind. If you are worried about your dreams discuss them with your doctor or midwife. Don't worry, nothing is too strange to report!

eclampsia Seizures occurring with severe hypertension brought on by pregnancy. They may occur after delivery. They can sometimes be prevented by intravenous medication but often occur without warning. Because most occur after delivery they do not affect the baby. If they occur before delivery urgent caesarean section may be required.

ectopic pregnancy Pregnancy outside the uterus usually occurs in a fallopian tube but rarely may occur on an ovary. It is usually associated with bleeding very early in the pregnancy and abdominal pain and is an extremely serious condition requiring immediate medical attention. In most institutions, the pregnancy is removed by laparoscopy (keyhole surgery) although a more formal operation may be required. It is usual to remove the tube where the pregnancy is. This does not reduce your fertility by 50 per cent, rather by a figure closer to 10 per cent. Diagnosis is usually on the basis of clinical examination, ultrasound and blood tests in early pregnancy. Before six weeks from the first day of your last period, it is rarely possible to see anything on ultrasound. Because some crampy pain is not unusual in early pregnancy the combination of light bleeding or spotting and some pain is unlikely to represent an ectopic pregnancy. If you have any bleeding very early on you should see a doctor to rule it out. Attendance at a maternity unit is the only way to clarify the issue definitively. If you have had an ectopic pregnancy you are more likely to have one again.

effacement The term used to describe the shortening of the cervix. In a first labour, the cervix effaces before beginning to dilate. If you have already had a baby, the cervix may efface and dilate at the same time.

embolus An embolus is a blood clot that travels usually from the leg or pelvis to the lungs. If it is small, it may merely cause chest pain and/or breathlessness. If very large, it may be fatal. There is an increased chance of developing an embolus with caesarean delivery. Treatment is by anticoagulation— thinning of the blood by injection or tablets. An amniotic fluid embolus is a rare event with a high rate of maternal death. It usually occurs around the time of delivery and is a grave medical emergency.

engagement When the baby's head has 'dropped' into the pelvis, or engaged, this usually signifies that the mother can have a successful vaginal delivery. Engagement usually occurs any time from week 36 onwards in a first pregnancy and later in a subsequent one.

engorgement The medical term used to describe when breasts are overly full of milk because milk is being produced that is not being excreted. If you do not breastfeed you can expect your breasts to become engorged after delivery. This may be very uncomfortable but will settle in 24–48 hours. Pills to suppress lactation are no longer given because they have been proven to be no more effective than sugar tablet placebos and there are some rare side effects associated with them. If you are breast-feeding and become engorged when you miss a feed, simply feed your baby or express as soon as you feel full because although the condition itself is not dangerous it can lead to mastitis.

'I felt like I was going to explode the morning after my milk came in. I had slept for about six hours without feeding and my breasts were almost twice their normal size. I fed immediately and that took some of the pressure off but every couple of hours they would fill up and start to leak. For a few nights I woke up doing the backstroke and was desperate to feed. Everything settled down after a couple of days.'

epidural anaesthetic A very popular form of pain relief given by passing a fine needle into one of the spaces surrounding the spinal cord, through which a numbing dose of local anaesthetic is administered. It may be topped up periodically. If you elect to have this kind of pain relief, you will require intravenous fluids, a urinary/bladder catheter and your mobility will be restricted. You may also be at increased risk of forceps/vacuum delivery or caesarean section.

'I had the epidural when I was 4 cm dilated and it was great for numbing the pain but it more or less seemed to stop my progress for a few hours. By the time things picked up it was beginning to wear off so I had a top up. My right side was definitely number than the left which felt very weird and I had to be told when to push because although I felt pressure on my stomach I didn't feel like pushing. I'm glad I had it on my first because there was so much going on and I was afraid of not being able to cope with the pain. I really hated having the catheter though and now that I know what to expect I'd like to try and have my next baby without an epidural.'

episiotomy A surgical cut made to enlarge the vaginal opening to allow the baby's head out, which requires stitches after delivery. Massaging almond oil and/or vitamin E into the perineum regularly in the latter half of pregnancy may reduce your chances of an episiotomy. The incidence of episiotomy varies from hospital to hospital. If you inquire about hospital rates, make sure the figure you are given is the number of episiotomies per vaginal births for first time mothers, and not all births (including caesareans) or the statistics may be misleading.

Erb's palsy A rare condition in a baby affecting his or her arm; it is usually due to damage to the baby's neck nerves following the complication of shoulder dystocia at delivery. Most cases recover by themselves during the first year of life but a small proportion of children are left with a variable degree of permanent disability.

ergometrine A medicine given by injection to assist with delivery of the placenta. It causes the uterus to contract and reduces the amount of blood lost at delivery.

expressing A term describing milking your own breasts. If you are having difficulty feeding your baby because of cracked nipples, your baby is in the special care unit or if you need to store milk for someone else to feed your baby with, you will need to milk yourself, or express milk. This is best achieved with an electric breast pump. Other methods take far too long and are difficult to master.

external cephalic version The technique for turning a breech baby to head first. It will usually be attempted after week 36 if your baby is bottom down. You may be given an injection to relax your uterus before the doctor coaxes the baby into the correct position by pressing down on your stomach from the outside. The risks (rupture of the membranes, separation of the placenta, foeto-maternal transfusion) associated with the procedure are extremely small.

external foetal monitoring The baby's heart rate is monitored by attaching a sensor disc to your abdomen with a big belt which traces the foetal heartbeat. Results are charted automatically onto paper, which can then be analysed by medical staff.

eye care Your prescription for contact lenses or glasses may change during pregnancy due to fluid retention that affects your own lens.

face presentation A clinical situation in labour where your baby's face, rather then the top of the head, is coming first through your pelvis. A caesarean section will usually be performed in this case, especially if the labour slows, although vaginal delivery is frequently possible without risk even if the baby's face is coming first.

fallopian tubes There are two fallopian tubes, one on each side of the uterus. Their purpose is to collect the egg and waft it towards the uterus. Fertilisation normally takes place in one tube but if the pregnancy implants there, it is ectopic and cannot progress.

false labour Transient episodes of painful uterine contractions which make you think you are going into labour. If your cervix has not started the changes associated with labour (effacement and dilatation) the contractions don't represent true labour, but rather are a false alarm.

fatigue Fatigue comparable to jet lag that will not go away is a common complaint in the first half of pregnancy. It usually lifts around week 18 or 20. Only rarely is it associated with anemia.

fibroids Benign swellings in the uterus, or fibroids, often grow during pregnancy and may obstruct delivery if they are in the lower part of the uterus. They may cause considerable pain during pregnancy. They may also very rarely cause miscarriage. It is often best to have them surgically removed before getting pregnant.

'My pregnancy was pretty tough because I had large fibroids that really, really hurt all the time and more so as the baby got bigger. I had difficulty working and going out and had to take it really easy because I was permanently worn out. I didn't want to complain too much though because the pain was the least of my worries and my doctor said nothing could be done about it. I was so nervous that I would have a miscarriage. I wish I had gone to the doctor before I got pregnant because even then I had really painful periods and maybe something could have been done at that stage.'

first stage of labour The part of labour when the cervix dilates, or opens, from being closed to 10 cm (full dilatation).

foetal monitoring In labour the term refers to listening to your baby's heart. It can be done either with a special stethoscope or electronically by a machine. A special clip attached to the baby's scalp during a pelvic examination in labour can feed information about the baby's pulse rate into an electronic monitor. The technique is very widely used although its use is not associated with any improved long term outcome for the baby and is associated with a higher rate of operative deliveries—caesareans or vacuum/forceps delivery.

foeto-maternal haemorrhage This occurs when a baby bleeds into the mother's blood stream through the placenta. It can occur spontaneously, when it may be associated with a non-specific feeling of being unwell or shivering, or it can occur after a blow to the abdomen, amniocentesis or (rarely) external cephalic version. It may be a sudden rapid event in which case the baby may die, or it may be gradual when intervention may be life-saving for the baby. If gradual, it may be associated with a reduction in foetal movements. It is diagnosed by a Kleihauer blood test.

foetoscopy A small tubular light and strong lens is inserted into the uterus similarly to cordocentesis so that the baby can be visualised. It is used only in exceptional circumstances, in only a few hospitals in the world (*see* **laser**).

folic acid A dietary supplement, only proven to improve the baby's health if taken prior to conception and for the first trimester, folic acid is found in green leafy vegetables and most fortified commercial breads and breakfast cereals. It is advisable to take folic acid supplements if you are considering pregnancy.

follicle A small cyst-like structure in the ovary whence the egg is discharged at ovulation. A new follicle is formed each time ovulation occurs. Normally only one follicle develops in each menstrual cycle. Several may develop if you are taking fertility treatment.

fontanelle A soft spot at the top of the baby's head. In a newborn baby, the bones of the skull are not completely fused together so there is a soft spot at the top of its head. Although it seems delicate—you can often see it pulsing—it is tough enough to protect your baby's brain.

forceps Metal instruments placed either side of the baby's head that are used to assist in delivery of the baby if you have difficulty pushing or your baby appears to be in distress. Forceps are uncommon in second and subsequent births.

forewaters Amniotic fluid lying in front of your baby's head. Sometimes this will leak for a while and then stop in late pregnancy (*see* **hindwaters**).

fundus The top of the uterus. The distance between the fundus and pubic bone roughly corresponds in centimetres to the number of weeks you are pregnant. Its measurement may therefore be noted at each antenatal visit.

gas (pain relief) A mixture of oxygen and nitrous oxide. During the active stage of labour, it is possible to get some pain relief from inhaling this gas, which is self-administered. As a contraction begins, you simply inhale deeply until the contraction has peaked. If you get the timing right and don't depend on the gas for too long, the relief is considerable. It also provides a welcome distraction. Some women say however that the gas makes them feel ill and disorientated.

genes The proteins that determine and direct bodily development and functions. Genes are collected together into groups known as chromosomes. Half of a baby's genes come from the mother and half from the father.

glucose challenge test A preliminary test for diabetes in which fewer samples are taken than in a glucose tolerance test. It is usually done before a glucose tolerance test.

glucose tolerance test A test for diabetes involving a series of blood tests in which blood sugar levels are measured.

group B streptococcus (GBS) GBS is an organism (bug) that is present in up to 30 per cent of women and may cause an infection in the newborn baby. If an infection has occurred in the past, or if you are in a high-risk group for infection, you will be prescribed an antibiotic in labour. Taking this antibiotic will almost eliminate the chances of your baby developing an infection. High risk cases include prematurity and rupture of membranes 24 hours before labour. Antenatal screening for GBS is not done routinely.

haemorrhage (*see also* **lochia; antepartum, foeto-maternal** and **post partum haemorrhage**) The medical term for bleeding. It does not imply heavier bleeding than when the term 'bleeding' is used. Antepartum haemorrhage is bleeding before birth; post-partum haemorrhage is bleeding after birth.

haemorrhoids (*see* **piles**)

hair loss (alopecia) You may find that your hair thins considerably after delivery or after you stop breastfeeding. This may very occasionally happen during pregnancy, but in any case is only temporary.

hare lip *see* **cleft or hare lip and palate**

headache You may be more susceptible to headaches during pregnancy, which hardly seems fair given that pregnant women should try to avoid painkillers. The headaches are usually the result of hormonal changes and the increased blood volume characteristic of pregnancy but may be intensified by stress, hunger and fatigue—all of which you should strive to control as much as possible. If your headache is accompanied by fever and flu symptoms or it persists, paracetamol is recommended over aspirin and ibuprofen.

heartburn A burning sensation in your lower chest or upper abdomen due to acid indigestion. As pregnancy hormones relax the muscles around the valve between your oesophagus and stomach and the uterus pushes up on the stomach, acid from the junction between the stomach and oesophagus can back up towards the throat causing an unpleasant burning sensation. Antacids, which are usually full of calcium (a bonus), can be taken in moderation to help alleviate symptoms. Otherwise, all you can do is eat less more often, avoid spicy foods and sleep slightly upright. Occasionally, your doctor may prescribe a tablet to cut down on acid production in your stomach.

heel prick test A test administered to babies a few days after birth to test for PKU, cystic fibrosis and other inborn errors of metabolism which, if left untreated, can cause serious illness in your baby.

HELLP syndrome A variant of toxaemia (pre-eclampsia), HELLP stands for Hypertension Elevated Liver enzymes Low Platelets. Diagnosis is made based on a blood sample and treatment is delivery of the baby.

Heparin A drug given by injection to thin the blood if there has been a clot in the veins. It is safe for the baby.

hindwaters The amniotic fluid behind the baby's head. Even if your hindwaters leak before labour you may still need your forewaters broken in labour.

hirsutism Excessive hair growth. Some women find that their facial and body hair growth increases during pregnancy and for a few months afterwards. Unwanted hair is best removed by waxing or non-chemical methods as skin can be ultrasensitive during pregnancy and post partum (the period after the birth).

HIV (human immunodeficiency virus) An infectious disease usually transmitted by the use of infected needles when abusing drugs, by engaging in promiscuous sexual activity, particularly if there is any break in the skin or via contaminated blood transfusion. Most countries screen for HIV in pregnancy because if a mother is positive her baby can be protected by her receiving appropriate treatment. An untreated mother can transfer the infection to her child.

hydatidiform mole Abnormal development of the placenta where it forms as a mass of grape-like cysts. It occurs in approximately one in 2,000 pregnancies, particularly in women over 45. With no placenta to support it, the fertilised ovum deteriorates. Symptoms of a molar pregnancy are severe morning sickness, a brownish vaginal discharge and a larger than normal uterus. The ovaries may also be enlarged. A d&c is necessary and conscientious follow-up monitoring of hormone levels as up to 15 per cent of molar pregnancies fail to stop growing even after the d&c. Sometimes a second d&c, and occasionally medication, is required followed by monitoring of blood beta HCG levels. The condition is often diagnosed by ultrasound but may only be apparent when tissue removed at the time of d&c for miscarriage is examined under the microscope.

hydrocephalus A potentially fatal condition where there is excess fluid in the brain cavities. It is often associated with other neurological malformations such as spina bifida.

hyperemesis Excessive vomiting in pregnancy. Although rare, excessive vomiting resulting in dehydration and fatigue, requires hospitalisation for rehydration. The condition may persist throughout pregnancy although it most commonly subsides by week 12. If you vomit more than three times a day for three days or if absolutely nothing (including fluids) is staying down, notify your doctor. Hyperemesis will have no effect on your baby.

'I had mild morning sickness in the beginning and then it got really bad soon after my first antenatal visit. I could barely keep from gagging when I drank water, let alone food. I lost a few pounds one week and had absolutely no energy so I went to see my GP because I wasn't due for another antenatal appointment for weeks. She immediately got in touch with the hospital and I had to be admitted. I stayed in for three days and went back in twice more after that. Later in the pregnancy, my nausea improved but I didn't feel enthusiastic about food until after the baby was born.'

hysterectomy Removal of the uterus. It may be necessary after delivery on very rare occasions if haemorrhage cannot be controlled by any other treatment. It is rarely necessary, although it is more frequent after a previous caesarean section because the placenta may develop at the site of the scar and may cause bleeding after delivery. It is very unlikely that the ovaries would also be removed.

incontinence Involuntary passage of urine or faeces. Many women find it difficult to control their bladder functions during pregnancy while others find that muscle damage during childbirth has affected their control of both bladder and bowel. Leaking urine when laughing or coughing is a common and potentially embarrassing complaint in late pregnancy and for some women for years after they have given birth. A strong pelvic floor toned by exercise can help prevent incontinence. Before and after delivery, simply tighten your anal and vaginal muscles as tightly as you can as if trying not to urinate, hold for 8–10 seconds, then release slowly while standing or sitting. Try to do 25 repetitions in the course of the day. If you experience leaking in the anus or back passage, inform your doctor.

induction The process of starting labour artificially. If your baby is overdue or you suffer from hypertension, pre-eclampsia, heart disease, diabetes or bleeding or there are signs that the placenta is not functioning properly, labour may be induced. Prostaglandin pessaries, inserted in the vagina may trigger labour over the following hours. Sometimes an oxytocin intravenous drip is used instead. Most often, the waters are broken in hospital. The doctor inserts an instrument not unlike a long crochet hook into the vagina and punctures the amniotic sac with it, causing the waters to drain. There can be a gush of warm liquid or a surprisingly small amount of fluid drained but in either case, although generally not painful, amniotomy is not the most pleasant of procedures. Labour usually starts soon after it is performed (within hours).

insomnia Inability to sleep. In the run-up to birth, few women sleep through the night. You may find that though you are physically tired your mind races when you lie down to go to sleep. Perhaps this is nature's way of training mothers to cope with the nocturnal demands of their children! In any case, it is normal in late pregnancy to get up a few times during the night because it is difficult to find a comfortable sleeping position or because you need to empty your bladder. Alternatively, you may have disturbing dreams, foot and leg cramps or heartburn. You may even have all of the above. No matter how hard you find it, try to avoid sleeping pills unless prescribed by your doctor to break a cycle of sleeplessness. Medications can cross the placenta to the baby.

intertrigo A red rash found in sweaty skin folds, usually under the breasts and in the groin. Irritating skin rashes are common in pregnancy—when the belly stretches, the skin often becomes dry and itchy. Most common in overweight women, the condition can be avoided or controlled by limiting weight gain, bathing frequently and gently powdering the affected areas. Calamine lotion may also help; hydrocortisone ointments, which thin the skin,

should only be used following consultation with your doctor.

involution The return of the uterus to normal size following pregnancy. It is usually complete within six weeks of delivery.

jaundice (*see also* **bilirubin**) The yellow discolouration of the skin due to bilirubin. In the newborn it is due to a breakdown of foetal blood cells during the transition period after birth and is usually self limiting ie it resolves itself. In pregnant women it may be due to slowing down in the gall bladder and liver or to a variety of infections. There may be associated itchiness of the skin due to bile pigments irritating the skin. If you feel you are jaundiced, bring it to the attention of your caregivers.

Kell antibodies Unusual antibodies in the blood that may cause anemia in a baby (*see* **rhesus disease** and **anti D**).

Kleihauer test A blood test on the mother for the presence of foetal cells in her circulation.

labia The fleshy lips of tissue at the entrance to the vagina.

lanugo The fine downy hair that covers the foetus from week 16 until term, when it begins to disappear. Most babies still have some lanugo left on their shoulders, face and backs when they are born.

laser Laser treatment of identical twins is sometimes indicated if there is evidence of abnormal communication of blood vessels between the twins—twin to twin transfusion syndrome. The communicating vessels are 'zapped' with the laser.

latching on refers to the baby attaching itself to the breast for feeding. Hungry babies will attack with great gusto and need to be steered to the proper position so they take the full areola into their mouths when they latch on.

let down reflex A complex reflex triggered by the baby sucking at the breast. It starts the flow of milk within a few seconds. Some mothers can actually feel it happening and experience a tingling feeling in their neck where the pituitary gland is or a more generalised sense of relief as the milk begins to flow. Proper positioning of the baby's mouth around the areola facilitates the whole process.

libido Sexual appetite. Many women find that their sexual appetite decreases during pregnancy. In the beginning, nausea and an unfounded fear of damaging the foetus may put some women off. Others find that during the first three months, they are more easily aroused. Later, sex may be physically uncomfortable or you may be too tired to enjoy it. Men's attitudes towards their partners also vary throughout pregnancy and after the birth. Simply put, some men find a bulging belly attractive, others don't. For a few weeks, or even months, following the birth, most couples find themselves preoccupied with the new baby or too exhausted to contemplate anything but sleep. They may also be apprehensive about intercourse being painful after stitches. After the big event, it naturally takes time for things to settle back down to normal. Both parties need to be especially aware and tolerant of each other's fluctuating feelings and sensitivities.

'Having a long session is the last thing I feel like right now (I'm 34 weeks). I feel like a beached whale. I can't believe anybody would want to sleep with me but I feel sorry for my husband so we do make love once a week or so. I feel like my body knows the act is redundant.'

lightening When the baby's head engages in the pelvis (for first mothers this usually happens in the month preceding delivery), you may be relieved to feel much less pressure on your upper abdomen, or a lightening.

linea nigra A straight, dark line, or linea nigra, begins to appear between the belly button and the pubis around week 14 as skin pigmentation around the nipples also begins to darken. In sallow skinned women, the line can be very pronounced and may not disappear for up to a year after delivery. The line has no significance to mother or child. Not every woman develops a linea nigra and whether you do or don't has no implications for your baby.

liquor The fluid in the amniotic sac where the baby grows and develops. It is usually clear, certainly up until the end of pregnancy, and is produced by both the placenta and the baby. Most of the liquor in the last three months is produced by the baby's kidneys although some is produced by the lungs. Liquor provides a warm, shock absorbent environment for your baby's growth and exercise. It is body temperature, which is why newborn babies usually cry after birth— they're cold! Imagine stepping out of a hot shower into a cold room. A normal volume of fluid at the end of pregnancy is a good sign for your baby. The amount of fluid may be assessed by ultrasound if there is any doubt or if you are overdue.

listeria An organism that can infect a baby in the womb causing a congenital pneumonia, which may be fatal. Listeria is found in foods that are likely to be in and out of the fridge in warm weather, such as salads, chicken, pâté, soft cheeses. If you eat freshly cooked foods it is unlikely you will be at risk. Listeria may cause only a flu-like illness in you or may have no effect at all, thus making it difficult to diagnose. As a cause of foetal death it is rare.

lochia Vaginal discharge following delivery. The amount and colour of the lochia reflect the degree of involution, or shrinkage, of the uterus. Immediately after the birth it is bright red and quite profuse. You may pass a few small blood clots, particularly during the strong uterine contractions that occur during breastfeeding. Usually after the fourth day, the colour changes to a reddish brown, then to brown. When you become more active, it may turn red again but ultimately it turns a pink or yellowish brown with intermittent red periods until it ceases altogether. Breastfeeding is often associated with sporadic periods of red bleeding for anything from 14 days to eight weeks. The average is about three weeks. If you are concerned about the amount of bleeding you are experiencing, contact your doctor or hospital.

LS ratio (lecithin sphingomyelin ratio) The ratio of two chemicals secreted by the baby's lungs into the amniotic fluid may be measured if premature delivery is being considered in either the baby's or mother's interests. If the ratio is greater than 2:1 it suggests the baby's chances of developing respiratory distress are minimal. The test requires amniocentesis to collect amniotic fluid. If delivery is expected in days or weeks, it may be recommended to give steroids to stimulate the baby's lung maturity and lessen the chances of foetal respiratory problems. The test is rarely done nowadays.

luteinising hormone (LH) The hormone secreted before ovulation; home ovulation kits test for its presence in the urine.

mastitis A breast infection, or mastitis, which can be caused by germs getting into a cracked nipple during breastfeeding, should be treated as quickly as possible to prevent it developing into an abcess. You can develop mastitis without a cracked nipple, however, and not every woman with a cracked nipple gets mastitis. If you suffer from a fever, localised redness, swelling, flu-like aches, nausea and vomiting, see a doctor immediately. Once treated with antibiotics, the infection usually begins to subside in 24 hours. You should feed through the illness even if it is painful. Doing so will not harm your baby but it will help you. The infection is in your breast, not your milk, and not feeding will only lead to engorgement and possibly blocked milk ducts or abcess formation.

meconium The dark green, almost black intestinal secretion the baby normally passes after birth is the consistency of tar. While still in the uterus, the baby also passes meconium (more and more as term approaches), which is absorbed into the amniotic fluid. During labour the presence or absence of meconium in the amniotic fluid is noted as it can be an indication of the health of the baby.

mid trimester bleed Bleeding which occurs between weeks 12 and 24 is often described as a mid trimester bleed because it occurs in the middle part of pregnancy before the foetus is viable—able to survive outside the womb. Such bleeding is not common but if it happens repeatedly the chances of premature delivery increase, especially if there is associated pain and contractions.

miscarriage A pregnancy that ends before week 24 is considered a miscarriage. One third of all pregnancies end in miscarriage in the first few weeks of pregnancy, a quarter of these before pregnancy has even been confirmed. Most of these happen because of foetal abnormalities. The chance of miscarrying increases with age and the number of your previous pregnancies. If you experience any bleeding during your pregnancy, you should consult your doctor immediately. Regardless of when in the pregnancy miscarriage occurs, it can be a profoundly upsetting experience for mothers and fathers alike and must be handled sensitively. For more information contact the Miscarriage Association of Ireland, Carmichael Centre, North Brunswick Street, Dublin 7, tel (01) 873 5702, 872 5550, 872 2914 www.carmichaelcentre.ie

molar degeneration (hydatidiform mole) may also be associated with excessive pregnancy symptoms, particularly vomiting. This is a rare condition in which the placenta degenerates into a mass of small grape-like cysts, which produce excessive amounts of HCG.

mole A dark skin patch, like a freckle. If you have a mole, it is likely it will darken during pregnancy because of general changes in pigmentation. If you notice growth or bleeding or you are concerned, show it to your doctor.

mood changes Every prospective or new mother is at one time or another given to mood changes. Bear with them. If you are unable to cope, or crying all the time for no apparent reason, you may be suffering from depression. Don't be afraid to seek help.

morning after pill If taken within 48–72 hours of intercourse, the MAP is felt to reduce the chances of becoming pregnant. Usually, the MAP is more than one pill—several high dose oral contraceptives, which are taken in two doses 12 hours apart. The medication may make you feel nauseous or you may vomit and have some vaginal bleeding. The pills are most easily available from your GP or a family planning clinic.

morning sickness Nausea can occur at any time day or night so the term 'morning sickness' is a misnomer. During pregnancy, most women are prone to nausea—for most it will end around week 12–14. It may return again in late pregnancy or persist throughout if you are unlucky. The presence or absence of nausea has no bearing on the baby's health and is no indication of your baby's sex. The best way to ward off nausea is by eating smaller meals more often so your stomach is never completely empty nor too full. Some scientists believe that nausea is nature's way of limiting exposure to certain toxins in the diet and environment.

Moro reflex Babies are born with a number of instinctual reactions to stimuli. For example, if startled, a young infant will throw its arms and legs out suddenly and clench its fists before relaxing again. The paediatrician will check the baby for the presence of this standard Moro reflex.

moulding Refers to the shape of the baby's head at birth. A baby's skull bones are soft and not joined together so it can squeeze into different positions during birth. Once engaged, the skull may mould to the shape of the birth canal—this is a normal physio-logical event. The baby's head will regain its normal shape within a few days of birth.

mucous plug A plug of mucus that blocks the cervix during pregnancy. Prior to the onset of labour, the mucus lodged at the opening of the uterus usually comes away. It may also be dislodged by a pelvic exam. Labour may not start right away or even for weeks but the loss of the plug is usually a sign that the cervix has begun to thin and ripen.

multigravida/multiparous A woman who has had at least one baby.

multiple pregnancy More than one baby in a pregnancy. The most common type of multiple pregnancy is twins. The more babies a woman is carrying, the greater the potential for complications. Non-identical twins have a lower rate of complications than identical twins. Fertility treatment is often associated with multiple pregnancy.

myomectomy The removal of a fibroid. The procedure is rarely, if ever, done in pregnancy or at time of caesarean because of the risk of haemorrhage.

nasal congestion A feeling of the nose being partly blocked. The mucous membranes of the nose swell and soften during pregnancy as the blood circulation increases. This may lead to stuffiness and/or nosebleeds that only stop occurring after delivery. If you are prone to nosebleeds, try not to blow your nose too vigorously. To stop the bleeding, lean forward slightly and apply gentle pressure just below the bridge of your nose.

nausea (*see* **morning sickness**)

nipples When breastfeeding, the whole nipple and areola surrounding it must be placed well inside the baby's mouth. Even still, the nipples can be susceptible to painful cracking and bleeding. To protect them, expose them to air between feeds and if necessary, wear a light plastic nipple shield during feeding for a day or two to ease the initial pain of the baby's sucking. Cracks will heal quickly if some of the colostrum or milk from the breast is gently rubbed into them with a clean fingertip. If the breasts leak, breast pads should be changed frequently so that soured milk does not find its way into cracks and cause infection.

nuchal translucency Refers to a pad of tissue at the back of the baby's head. In early pregnancy (between 11 and 13 weeks) an ultrasound scan can assess the thickness of this pad. If the pad is thicker than normal there is an increased risk of Down syndrome.

The test is a 'marker' and is not diagnostic of Down syndrome in itself.

occipito-posterior position The baby's head is in the face up position rather than the usual face down position. During labour, the baby's head normally rotates as it passes through the birth canal so that usually by the time of delivery the baby is facing the mother's back passage and the top of the head is facing forwards. In about 10 per cent of cases, however, the baby's head rotates to face forward and the top of the head (occiput) is facing back (posterior). Most of the time, this causes no problems and does not interfere with labour or delivery. It may however, result in more low back pain during labour and require assistance in delivery (rarely, a caesarean may be necessary). It is not a serious problem and its importance is frequently overstated. The position of the baby's head before labour is of no consequence whatsoever.

oedema Swelling of the ankles, feet and hands, or oedema is to be expected to some degree. Extreme swelling is another matter and should be mentioned to your doctor. Water retention is exacerbated by too much salt in the diet, too much weight gain, too much standing and hot weather. Severe oedema may require hospitalisation for observation but this is very rare. Putting your feet up will reduce ankle swelling by redistributing fluid but it will reappear when you are upright again. There is no way of getting rid of retained fluid during pregnancy. It will recede naturally after delivery. Ankle and feet oedema is very common in the first week or so after delivery if you have received a lot of fluid during labour because, for example, you had an epidural or caesarean section.

oxytocin (pitocin) The natural hormone excreted by the pituitary gland that stimulates labour is sometimes given intravenously to induce or accelerate labour.

partograph A graph used to plot your progress in labour.

perinatal The term used to describe the time around birth. A perinatal death refers to any baby who is stillborn or who dies in the first four weeks of life. The perinatal death rate is generally 1 per cent or less in the Western world. (In other words, if a baby reaches 24 weeks or 500 g weight it has a greater than 99 per cent chance of survival.)

perineum The area between the vagina and the rectum. It should be able to stretch adequately during birth to allow the baby to emerge. If it is not elastic enough, the perineum may tear, requiring stitches, or an episiotomy may be performed. Pelvic floor exercises (*see* **incontinence**) will help strengthen the area and improve its flexibility and should be done throughout pregnancy.

pethidine Morphine-based narcotics like pethidine can be injected into the thigh or buttock during labour to provide pain relief. Pethidine can make you feel dizzy and disorientated even in small doses. In large doses, it can sedate the baby.

phantom pregnancy A very rare condition in which a woman convinces herself she is pregnant and exhibits all the symptoms of pregnancy including a swollen abdomen. Once pregnancy is excluded with an ultrasound scan (the widespread availability of which has made the condition less common), the condition requires psychiatric treatment.

piles Varicose veins in the rectum (haemorrhoids) often plague women in late pregnancy (particularly if they have already had a baby), and afterwards, in the postpartum. The pressure of the growing baby on the rectum coupled with constipation or straining and increased progesterone levels cause this unpleasant condition as can the strain on the area during labour and delivery. Bleeding is common, particularly after a bowel motion and sometimes, the piles may become so large they protrude outside the anus. Over-the-counter ointments may help reduce swelling or your doctor may prescribe a local anaesthetic ointment to help ease the pain. More rarely, a pile becomes extremely swollen and sore (thrombosed) and can be felt as a small, round, hard area. This will be very painful and uncomfortable for about three days and then will begin to disappear of its own accord. Very rarely, a thrombosed pile needs to be operated on during pregnancy. Treatment for prolapsed piles is not recommended until after delivery when they can be injected or operated upon. All you can do in the meantime is take a warm bath and gently push them back in. Untreated piles will return and be worse in subsequent pregnancies so it is well worth trying to avoid them in the first place by eating a high fibre diet and avoiding lifting heavy weights in late pregnancy. In most cases when piles

occur it is because they are unavoidable and not due to anything you may have done or not done.

PKU (phenylketonuria) A rare condition present from birth due to an enzyme deficiency, PKU is treated with a special diet. Left untreated, it will result in mental retardation. PKU and other inborn errors of metabolism are tested for in the heel prick test administered a few days after birth.

placenta (afterbirth) The incredibly versatile organ that supports the foetus and reaches maturity around week 34. It acts as the baby's lungs, kidneys and bowel and produces several hormones. At term it weighs approximately one sixth of the baby's weight.

placenta praevia The placenta is normally found in the upper part of the uterus. In 1 per cent of pregnancies it is situated in the lower part of the uterus, below the baby's head instead of above it, which almost always causes some bleeding to occur in late pregnancy. Any bleeding that occurs after week 28 should be investigated to check for placenta praevia. The routine scan between weeks 18–20 will confirm the position of the placenta. If the condition is diagnosed after 28 weeks, you will probably be admitted to stay in hospital until delivery so that subsequent bleeds can be monitored. Circumstances vary greatly however so that care can be adjusted to suit the individual pregnancy. Placenta praevia requires delivery by caesarean section.

placental insufficiency If the placenta fails to function efficiently, the health of the baby is compromised and it will not grow properly.

Regular antenatal visits will confirm that all is working smoothly and that growth is progressing normally. When you are overdue, the placenta may not function as efficiently as before term. As a mother, your best indication that your baby is well is if you are feeling it move, at least 10 movements per day in later pregnancy. A sick baby doesn't move.

polyhydramnios An excessive amount of amniotic fluid; it is associated with diabetes, multiple pregnancy and some malformations of the baby. Usually, it does not bode ill for either mother or baby.

polyp Polyps are benign growths, not cancerous. Occasionally a small growth, or polyp, on the cervix may bleed and need to be removed.

post-natal depression Mild feelings of anxiety and depression are normal in the first couple of weeks following birth but prolonged emotional upset, fatigue, paranoia, lack of self confidence, lethargy and indifference to the new baby are symptomatic of full-blown post-natal depression. Support and expeditious psychiatric treatment are vital.

post mortem examination is an investigation into the cause of death by performing an autopsy. An autopsy involves inspection of the body and opening body cavities, removing the organs for detailed examination and retaining parts for more examination under a microscope or doing special time-consuming tests. It may not be possible to determine the cause of death without an autopsy.

post partum haemorrhage Abnormal bleeding after delivery is uncommon but serious. Profuse bleeding that soaks more than one pad an hour for more than a few hours, massive blood clots, foul-smelling lochia or abdominal pain and swelling a few days after delivery could be signs that the uterus is not involuting (returning to normal size) properly, perhaps because of infection. There are two types of post partum haemorrhage; primary occurs in the first 24 hours following birth, secondary thereafter. Contact your doctor or hospital if you are worried about your bleeding. If you are breastfeeding it's not uncommon for the bleeding to stop and start for up to eight weeks.

pre-eclampsia A dangerous form of high blood pressure peculiar to pregnancy, which is most common in first time mothers, pre-eclampsia (also called toxaemia), occurs in 5–10 per cent of all women. Signs include sudden excessive weight gain, high blood pressure and protein in the urine. Blurred vision, headaches, irritability and acute abdominal pain may occur in severe cases. Routine checks of blood pressure and urine at antenatal clinics ensure that the vast majority of cases are caught well before they jeopardise the health of mother or baby. Mild cases are usually admitted for observation and labour is induced as soon as the cervix ripens. Sometimes outpatient management is appropriate in mild cases. If the disease progresses, you will be given medication to prevent convulsions and you will need immediate delivery.

prematurity Babies born before week 37 are defined as premature and may require special care although babies born as early as 26 weeks now have an excellent chance of survival. The closer to 37 weeks your baby is born the less likely special care will be needed.

primigravida A woman expecting her first baby.

progesterone A hormone secreted in large amounts during pregnancy, from the ovary in the very early stages and from the placenta after the first few weeks. There is no evidence that giving progesterone in early pregnancy reduces the chance of miscarriage. The only situation where it is medically indicated is in some cases of IVF pregnancy. If your progesterone level is low it is because there is a fundamental problem with your pregnancy. Giving extra progesterone will fix your blood level but not the underlying problem.

prolapse (cord) An uncommon condition where the umbilical cord comes through the cervix into the vagina and perhaps becomes visible outside it. It may cause death of the baby or severe foetal distress. If diagnosed in labour, it is usually associated with excellent outcome and has no long-term effects. It may be necessary for you to deliver by caesarean section.

prolapse (uterine) This may occur during or after pregnancy when the cervix and/or uterus descend into the vagina and sometimes protrude outside it. It is not dangerous but can be very uncomfortable. It usually improves within two to three months of delivery. Rarely, it may require surgery.

prostaglandins A group of chemicals which are used in obstetrics primarily to induce labour. A pessary of prostaglandin is inserted vaginally behind the cervix. The hoped for response is that the cervix will soften and open slightly (ripen) to allow rupture of the membranes (breaking the waters), or that labour itself will start (*see* **induction**).

ptyalism An excess of saliva, or ptyalism, is a harmless symptom of early pregnancy.

pubic symphysis The joint at the front of the pelvis where the pubic bones are joined by ligaments (*see* **symphysiotomy**). Slight separation may cause an intermittent, knife-like stabbing pain in the vagina late in pregnancy.

pudendal block If you don't have an epidural and need assistance with delivery (forceps or vacuum) your doctor may block the pudendal nerves, which will numb the area.

QFPCR stands for Qualitative Polymerase Chain Reaction. It is a genetic analysis which takes three days and detects a large number of major genetic abnormalities.

quickening The first perceptible foetal movements, referred to collectively as 'quickening' are noticeable between weeks 14–24. Experienced mothers may notice movement earlier than first-timers and thinner women may notice them earlier than heavier women.

recurrent miscarriage Three miscarriages in a row. If this happens, your doctor will suggest investigations to determine if possible what is causing them.

retroversion An unusual position of the uterus where it is leaning backwards, which occurs in about 15 per cent of women and is of no consequence. It has no effect on fertility and does not cause miscarriage. It may rarely block urination in early pregnancy necessitating admission to hospital for a day or two to drain the bladder.

rhesus disease (*see also* **anti D**) 15 per cent of Irish people lack a protein-like substance called the rhesus factor in their blood and are classified as rhesus negative. If a rhesus negative mother has a rhesus positive baby, she can become sensitised to the rhesus factor in the baby's blood so that her next pregnancy is at risk if that baby is also rhesus positive. An anti D injection will prevent the mother from forming rhesus antibodies.

ripening of the cervix The cervix, or neck of the womb, is firm and closed before labour begins and is often described as 'unripe'. At the beginning of labour the cervix becomes soft and slightly open before it begins to open progressively with advancing labour. This softening, or ripening, of the cervix can be artificially stimulated by medicines known as prostaglandins. This is often done in an attempt to induce labour, or start it artificially.

rooting Newborn babies will respond to the touching of their cheek by instinctively turning in the direction of the touch to feed. They are completely indiscriminate in their choice of targets and may root as furiously at a man's shirt sleeve as at their mother's breast.

round ligament pain Pain low on either side of the uterus can intensify as the uterus grows. This is similar to the pain of a strained Achilles tendon or hamstring muscle. It will ease with time and there is no specific treatment. Paracetamol may be taken for pain relief.

rubella or German measles may harm the foetus if the mother contracts it in early pregnancy. Most women are immune to Rubella as a result of childhood vaccination and your immune status will be checked routinely in early pregnancy. If you do get Rubella your baby is very unlikely to be affected in any way if you are further than 12 weeks into the pregnancy. In the first 12 weeks there is a risk of damage to the baby.

rupture of the membranes (*see also* **amniotomy**) When the waters break, or the membranes holding the amniotic fluid surrounding the baby are ruptured artificially, labour usually begins. The waters break spontaneously, before the onset of labour in about 30 per cent of all cases, and while the amount of fluid lost varies, it is usually more of a trickle than a flood because the baby's head blocks its flow.

sacro-iliac pain The classic, low backache of pregnancy may worsen with turning movements as simple as rolling over in bed. Massage, chiropractic manipulation or local heat may help ease any discomfort.

sciatica Sharp pains radiating down the lower back, buttocks and legs are not uncommon as pregnancy advances due to pressure on the sciatic nerve. The pains may come and go but nothing has been proven to help them. There is however a fair chance that you will wake in the morning after having been in considerable pain and it will have gone. Sciatica almost always goes away after delivery.

second stage of labour The part of labour from when the cervix is fully dilated to delivery of the baby.

shingles A painful condition which develops in people who have had chickenpox in the past. It is characterised by a rash along the line of a nerve, usually on the chest or face. It is not infectious.

shoulder dystocia An extremely uncommon event where the baby's shoulders get stuck after the baby' head has already been delivered. This is almost always unpredictable but is more common with very large babies and women with diabetes. After the baby's head has been born an attempt is made to deliver the baby's shoulders. The midwife and or doctor will manipulate the baby to effect delivery and during the course of this the baby's arms may be damaged. In most cases the baby is fine but in severe cases, there may be some paralysis or weakening of the baby's arm (Erb's palsy).

shoulder presentation The rare presentation of the baby's shoulder into the pelvis in labour requires caesarean delivery.

show One of the most common signs of the onset of labour is a bloody show, or discharge of mucus mixed with blood. Labour usually begins within 24 hours of the show. The show is often discharged at the same time as contractions begin.

SIDS *see* **sudden infant death syndrome**

skin problems Pigmentation darkens considerably during pregnancy. Some women find the T zone across their face is particularly affected when exposed to the sun (the so-called butterfly mask of pregnancy). Others experience acne for the first time in years or develop areas of itchiness and dryness. Little red spots (spider naevi—*see* **spider veins**) are not unusual on the chest and hands. They are little blood vessels grouped together and go pale when compressed. They are the result of hormonal stimulation and resolve after pregnancy.

skin tags Many women develop tiny skin tags, or little outcrops of skin, on the trunk during pregnancy, which usually disappear after delivery. They rarely need removal.

spider veins Purplish lines with a spidery aspect appear as a result of hormone changes. Unlike stretch marks, they can disappear after delivery. If they don't they can be removed later.

spina bifida A condition involving the spine, usually low down, which causes varying degrees of nerve damage and paralysis. It is the result of the spine not developing correctly in the very early stages of pregnancy. It is much less common now than in the past. The risk of spina bifida is very much reduced by taking folic acid supplements before pregnancy and in the early weeks. Anencephaly is the most severe form of spina bifida and is fatal, usually within hours of birth.

spinal anaesthetic Similar to an epidural but takes effect more quickly. It is usually used for caesarean section.

stillbirth Delivery of a dead baby after week 24 is characterised as a stillbirth. In almost one third of these cases, no cause of death is ever found. The physical effect on the mother is dramatic as the pregnancy hormones cease to be produced, resulting in weight loss and a waning of pregnancy symptoms. Suspicion is usually aroused because the baby stops moving. Labour usually begins within two or three days of the baby's death if the death has occurred close to the due date. Otherwise it is usual to induce the labour. This is an extremely traumatic experience and parents will need both sympathy and support during the birth and afterwards. A post mortem examination may reveal the cause of the death. A baby may look perfect on the outside but have a very significant internal abnormality that can only be detected by post mortem examination. Contact the Irish Stillbirth and Neonatal Death Society (ISANDS) (01) 872 6996 (01) 822 4688 www.carmichaelcentre.ie

stitches Perineal repairs after a natural tear or episiotomy during delivery are common on a first birth but increasingly less common on subsequent deliveries. As the wound heals, the stitches can become extremely uncomfortable. Good hygiene is crucial. Frequent baths help reduce the discomfort considerably and keep the area clean and free of infection. Exposure to air also helps. If sitting down is difficult, it may help to sit on a rubber ring. Modern stitches disintegrate and so do not need to be removed. They are sometimes slow to dissolve, however, taking up to four weeks in some cases. Don't put salt into the bath—it makes the stitches more painful and does not speed up healing. Soap and water are all you need.

stretch marks No amount of vitamin E cream or moisturiser can prevent stretch marks—the silvery indentations in the skin that accompany dramatic weight gain. Since most pregnancies are accompanied by a major weight gain, they are virtually unavoidable and the vast majority of women will develop at least a few marks. Although they will fade after delivery, they will never completely disappear.

sudden infant death syndrome (SIDS) The sudden death of an infant which remains unexplained after all known and possible causes have been excluded. The risk can be avoided by placing your baby on the back when sleeping (not face down), avoiding smoking around the baby, using a firm mattress and avoiding overheating the baby. Ninety per cent of babies who die from SIDS are under 6 months of age. Contact the Irish Sudden Infant Death Association 1850 391 391, (01) 873 2711 www.carmichaelcentre.ie

surfactant The chemical secreted by the baby's lungs in the uterus that prevents the lungs collapsing and the baby going into respiratory distress after birth. An artificial form of surfactant is available that can be given to premature babies. It is given by squirting the fluid directly down the baby's airways within minutes of birth.

symphysiotomy Spontaneous separation of the pubic symphysis may cause great pain but resolves itself soon after delivery as ligaments tighten up again.

teratogen Any substance that causes a foetal malformation, including alcohol and in the past, drugs like thalidomide and DES.

termination Termination is synonymous with induced abortion. Most terminations are undertaken for social reasons but some are performed because of foetal malformation or illness in the mother. They can be performed surgically, which is similar to d&c, or medically, usually by using prostaglandin to induce very premature labour.

third stage of labour The time from delivery of the baby until delivery of the placenta.

thrombosis (*see also* **embolus**) The formation of a clot, usually in a leg vein. Pregnancy predisposes to thrombosis.

thrush (monilia) More common in pregnancy, a candida infection or thrush, is aggravated by excess sugar in the system. Limit sugar intake and eat bio-yoghurt during an infection to help re-balance the vaginal flora. Also avoid tight fitting clothes. If the infection persists, you will need prescription medication. Even if you have an infection at the time of delivery it is very unlikely that your baby will be infected.

Thrush infection can occur in newborn babies even if you don't have an infection and it is rarely serious. An oral anti-fungal cream will clear the infection rapidly.

'After feeding, I noticed the inside of my baby's cheeks were coated in a white film, which I assumed was milk. When I tried to wipe it away with my finger it sort of peeled away and looked a bit like the skin that comes away after you burn your mouth. It didn't seem to bother her at all, though. I took her to the GP and he gave me a gel that sorted it out almost immediately.'

tocolytics Drugs given in an effort to stop premature labour. Considerable doubt exists as to their effectiveness.

toxaemia *see* **pre-eclampsia**

toxoplasmosis Undercooked meat, particularly poultry, and the faeces of infected animals, especially cats, carry a parasite that can be potentially dangerous to the foetus, causing blindness and brain damage. Most people have antibodies to the disease and so are immune to it, but in the early stages of pregnancy, you should avoid contact with raw meats and be careful around pets. You should not change litter boxes, poop scoop or garden with bare hands. Likewise, make sure all your food is well cooked.

transverse lie In a tiny percentage of pregnancies, the spine of the baby lies horizontal to the mother's. This is normally because the woman has had many previous pregnancies or because she is carrying excessive amniotic fluid. The baby can usually be manipulated into the proper position for birth. If it persists into labour caesarean section is necessary.

trimester A period of three months. Pregnancy is divided into three trimesters.

trisomy Chromosomes normally come in pairs; if a third chromosome attaches itself to the pair, the person carrying them will be affected by a serious genetic disorder. The most common trisomy is Down syndrome, or trisomy 21.

ultrasound An extremely common technique used to view the contents of the uterus. High frequency sound waves are directed into the body and are reflected back to a machine by bodily tissues. The results appear on a video screen. It can be used to estimate the age of the foetus, determine the number of foetuses and the position of the placenta, detect foetal abnormalities, diagnose miscarriage and later in pregnancy may be used to determine the health of the baby (*see* **biophysical profile**).

urinary tract infections Urinary tract infections affecting the bladder only are treated with antibiotics. If you have a severe infection accompanied by fever and vomiting, it will not harm the baby but may involve the kidneys so you may require hospitalisation for intravenous antibiotics. Trying to flush an infection out doesn't work and will only make you pee more often.

uterus (womb) The muscular organ that contains the developing foetus. The lower part, or outlet, is the cervix.

vacuum extraction A suction cup placed on the baby's head to assist delivery is felt to be associated with less damage to the perineum than forceps. Like forceps, it is unusual to need vacuum extraction in a second or subsequent delivery.

vaginal discharge Vaginal discharge normally becomes heavier during pregnancy. This is probably to prevent infection from ascending into the uterus. Discharge is frequently discoloured, often with a greenish tinge. As long as it isn't itchy or foul smelling, it is very unlikely to represent an infection. If you have a blood stained discharge, inform your doctor. A very watery discharge may be the result of rupture of the membranes.

varicose veins Swollen, prominent veins are the consequence of increased blood volume and the effect of muscle relaxing hormones. They are most common on the legs but may also occur on the vulva. Haemorrhoids are also a form of varicose veins. They often run in families and usually disappear after pregnancy. They will probably return in subsequent pregnancies so don't get your veins fixed or removed before your family is complete.

vernix The thick, waxy substance that covers the baby's skin to keep it from wrinkling in the womb. It diminishes in quantity if the baby is overdue.

viability Viability is the term used to describe the time after which the baby is capable of surviving independently, outside the womb. Although this time is defined as 24 weeks, in reality very few babies have a good chance of survival if they are born this early. Survival rates increase exponentially after 26 weeks.

visual disturbances You may get peculiar visual disturbances in pregnancy such as flashing lights before the eyes or blurred vision. These are of virtually no consequence but mention them to your doctor if they bother you. They are often associated with low blood pressure, which is normal in pregnancy.

vomiting In early pregnancy vomiting is usually due to hormonal changes. Sometimes in later pregnancy when your baby is pressing on your stomach it may make you vomit. Your stomach is also a lot more sensitive in pregnancy so even a mild dose of tummy upset that wouldn't bother you normally may make you vomit when you are pregnant. If your vomiting is so bad that not even fluids are staying down for a full day, you may need hydration in hospital. The vomiting will have no effect on your baby. Some women vomit in labour and often right after their baby is born, probably because of the sudden dropping of the stomach after delivery.

vulval varicosities Varicose veins in the vulva do not cause any problems with delivery. If you have them don't worry that they will bleed—they won't.

Warfarin A drug given to thin the blood when there has been a blood clot. It is not advised during pregnancy as it may cause a congenital abnormality (*see* **Heparin**).

yolk sac The small bit of tissue visible on very early ultrasound images, which is the source of nutrition for the embryo until the placenta develops.

zygocity refers to twin pregnancy. Monozygotic (identical) and dizygotic (fraternal/non identical) pregnancy is usually, but not always, detected by ultrasound.

zygote The very earliest description of the developing embryo before implantation.

useful contacts

For information on government services and entitlements, see www.oasis.gov.ie

AWARE—helping to defeat depression
www.aware.ie

Cuidiú—The Irish Childbirth Trust
www.cuidiu-ict.ie

Down Syndrome Ireland
www.downsyndrome.ie

Enable Ireland
www.enableireland.ie

Irish Multiple Birth Association
www.imba.ie

Irish Stillbirth and Neonatal Death Society (ISANDS)
www.isands.ie

Irish Sudden Infant Death Association (ISIDA)
www.isida.ie

La Lèche League
www.lalecheleagueireland.com

Miscarriage Association of Ireland
www.miscarriage.ie

Positive Options (+OPTIONS)
www.positiveoptions.ie

index